Cultural Competence

Edited by
Kathleen Kendall-Tackett, PhD, IBCLC, FAPA
& Scott Sherwood, BS

All royalties go to the
U.S. Lactation Consultant Association.

Praeclarus Press, LLC
©2015. United States Lactation Consultant Association

Praeclarus Press, LLC
2504 Sweetgum Lane
Amarillo, Texas 79124 USA
806-367-9950
www.PraeclarusPress.com

DISCLAIMER

The information contained in this publication is advisory only and is not intended to replace sound clinical judgment or individualized patient care. The author disclaims all warranties, whether expressed or implied, including any warranty as the quality, accuracy, safety, or suitability of this information for any particular purpose.

ISBN #978-1-939807-35-9

Cover Design: Ken Tackett

Acquisition & Development: Kathleen Kendall-Tackett & Scott Sherwood

Copy Editing: Kathleen Kendall-Tackett

Layout & Design: Nelly Murariu

Operations: Scott Sherwood

Contents

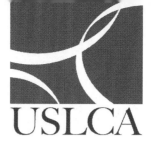

Working with Families of Different Cultures, Part I

Lessons Learned

Jeanette Panchula BSW, RN, PHN, IBCLC, RLC[1]

Keywords: Breastfeeding support, ethnic-group differences, cultural competence

The Code of Professional Conduct for IBCLCs states that an IBCLC must "Provide care to meet clients' individual needs that is culturally appropriate and informed by the best available evidence." IBCLCs must not only have knowledge that will help a mother breastfeed. They must also have the skill to help her to discern the best solution for her situation. The ability to communicate with clients does not necessarily mean learning "everything there is to know" about their culture. Rather, it means learning the basis for the mothers' beliefs and actions.

1   jeanette.panchula@sbcglobal.net

Looking back on 26 years as an IBCLC, and 36 years as a La Leche League Leader, I cannot imagine a more exciting, awe-inspiring, frustrating, and worthwhile career. I was raised in a multigenerational, bicultural, and bilingual household and city, San Juan, Puerto Rico. In San Juan, people of many different socioeconomic groups mixed in the market, the stores, and schools. As a result, I have always been comfortable with a variety of accents, beliefs, and ways of life. The concept that there is only one way—the way *I* was raised—was truly never expressed or taught to me. In fact, as a small child, I asked a nice man who was walking right by my porch: *Por qué tu eres tan negro?* [Why are you so black?]. Without missing a beat, he answered: *Porque estoy mucho al sol.* [Because I am in the sun a lot.]

That was the only education I received about race or skin color, as my parents did not believe it was an issue that I needed to be concerned with. It was only when a TV arrived in my home, and I saw horrible actions of others in the southern areas of the U.S. that I learned why my father would not move back to the U.S. with his dark-skinned, Puerto Rican wife, and very light-skinned (unless I spent a lot of time in the sun) daughter.

When I lived in St. Louis in the 80s with my own children, husband, and mother (she lived with us for 25 years)—I *did* experience how sales clerks and others *assumed* my mother was my maid. This preface is an explanation of why and how I arrived at the philosophy that I continue to practice today: All humans are different. All humans have their own story to tell. You cannot *look* at them and assume you know anything about them. You have to ask.

Assumption: Father is not involved/interested

You go into a hospital room, and you see a mother in the bed trying to breastfeed. She has a scarf over her head, keeping the hair out of her eyes as she works, and works at trying to get the baby on *right*. She is frustrated and worried. Her husband is on the other side of the curtain, at times reading a book, at times speaking to her, urging her to *try this* or *try that*. Then he goes back to reading.

Fact: Mom and dad are practicing orthodox Jews. Her head is covered as she should during the period that she is bleeding. She is untouchable at this time, and her husband is following strictly the instructions that he must not look at his wife's body during this time.

Actions: I stand in a location that allows both mother and father to see me. I use a doll to demonstrate positioning to both (this is prior to Biological Nurturing®). We then discuss how the father can help his wife by identifying where she can sit and be comfortable, what pillows she may need, what foods are comforting to her, and how to burp and change the baby. He was so relieved to know that he could do something instead of being vilified as an uninterested or demanding jerk.

How did we get there? By my asking: Can you tell me what you need? What are your concerns? What help will you be getting at home? This was the key. Both let me know about their beliefs: not the beliefs of *the Orthodox Jewish*, but *theirs*.) I have worked with people of many different religions, and know that what they do isn't just because they're Jewish or Catholic or Muslim or Protestant. What they do is because of how they *practice* their beliefs.

Assumption:
They won't accept information or instructions offered by someone of a different culture

I made a home visit with a Public-Health Nurse. We knew the mother was from Ethiopia and was Muslim. As the nurse was Jewish and I was Catholic, we both put the symbols we usually wear around our necks inside our blouses. No need to stress the mother with an obvious sign that may increase her concern about dealing with Americans!

Fact: When we arrived, she was already breastfeeding. It was obvious she was in pain and her baby was damaging her nipple. We also could see that he was very straight: unable to curve against her body in any way. Upon undressing the baby to weigh him, we found a very, very, very long piece of fabric had been wound around his torso from hips to under his arms.

Actions: We asked about this fabric, commenting that the colors and patterns were interesting. She said her mother had sent it to her from her country with instructions to wrap it around him to keep his back straight. We asked how she felt about it. She said she was not sure it was needed, but she didn't know whether she would be hurting her baby if she did not use it. We asked if it would be OK to not wrap the baby after weighing, and to try a different way to put the baby to the breast (again this was before BN). She looked relieved: *anything would be better than what I'm going through!* A much-better latch was achieved. And we provided additional information related to the value of allowing baby's own muscles and bones to achieve the desired straight back. During all follow-up visits it was evident the fabric was never used again.

How did we get there? By asking, being attentive to verbal and non-verbal cues, and then truthfully replying with information.

Assumption:
African American mothers
don't breastfeed

A mother delivered her baby in a local hospital. Nurses on the floor did not go in to ask about her breastfeeding: after all, she was African American. However, the IBCLC came on the floor and decided to ask them how they were doing.

Fact: They were doing very well. The mother, the grandmother, and the father had all attended a six-session training offered in their church for free. And they were all Peer Counselors for the A More Excellent Way Program (www.mewpeers.org).

Action: None needed, except educating the staff that yes, African American mothers do breastfeed when provided the right rationale at the right time with the right information and resources—and they have a family and community that supports them.

Question: Is that not the same for all mothers?

Assumption: Hispanic mothers do not exclusively breastfeed

Fact: Mothers in hospitals sometimes ask for formula. When the mother is Hispanic, many of the staff just sigh, often do not take the time to get on a translation line, or try to locate someone who speaks Spanish to provide information and education about the importance and value of exclusive breastfeeding because *they* always supplement.

Fact: Carol Melcher, RNC, CLE, MPH, together with the Perinatal Services Network of Loma Linda University in California, developed a program called Birth and Beyond (now evolved to Soft Hospital, http://carolmelcher.com/assets/soft_workbook.pdf). She was often told that some hospitals would never be able to achieve high exclusive breastfeeding rates because they had large Hispanic populations. The Birth and Beyond team created collaborations that resulted in 10 hospitals becoming Baby Friendly. This included hospitals primarily serving the Hispanic community. Part of the project included adding staff to help gather data and provide additional services. In this case, they hired someone who was knowledgeable about breastfeeding, and fluent in Spanish. She could then explain to parents the importance of early skin to skin, avoiding pacifiers and bottles, and all the other policies that were part of their hospital's maternity services in their own language. The outcome: hospitals serving primarily Hispanic mothers had exclusive breastfeeding rates that rose in the same way as hospitals serving non- Hispanic mothers.

Fact: Jane Heinig, PhD, IBCLC, RLC, and her team from the Human Lactation Center at UC Davis (http:// lactation.ucdavis.edu/aboutus/index.html), led focus groups of Hispanic mothers as a part of their research of infant feeding practices in the WIC program. She reported in the first California Breastfeeding Summit (2011) that *not one mother* in the focus groups stated that they requested formula *because my culture does it*. All mothers reported the same fears, concerns, insecurities, and frustrations that have been listed since research on the perceived barriers to breast-feeding began:

> » I don't think I'm doing it right.

> » He wants to eat all the time.

> » I don't have enough milk.

Action: Asking a mother—Hispanic, Asian, African American, or from anywhere—why she wants formula usually leads to identifying concerns common to all mothers. Ideally staff should be fluent and able to dialogue with the mother. However, many hospitals have limited number of staff fluent in Spanish (or the many other languages of the mothers they serve, especially in California). They may be able to communicate the basic information in a few sentences. But mothers who have concerns need more. They need to hear that *this is a very common worry mothers have,* and *we have people here and after discharge that can help you,* and *let me come by in a few minutes after you've tried xxx.*

When mothers are provided support by people who speak their language, they will accept the information. How this is done can vary.

> » Improving the knowledge about breast-feeding support to the staff that *is* fluent in other languages.

» Collaborating with local programs, such as WIC, to provide staff and/or peer counselors to support breastfeeding mothers in and out of the hospital. Linking mothers to groups and agencies that have staff that speak her language.

» Inviting local community agency staff to any breastfeeding trainings offered in hospitals or community centers.

You can find more specific information on communication skills in working with families from different cultures in Panchula (2012b).

Clinical Lactation, 2012, Vol. 3-1, 13-15

Reference

Panchula, J. (2012b). Working with families of different cultures II: Improving our communication skills. *Clinical Lactation*, 3(1), 16-20

Resources for Further Studies

Journal of Transcultural Nursing, Thousand Oaks, CA: Sage Publications

Health Resources and Services Administration (HRSA): *Indicators of cultural competence in health care delivery organizations: An organizational cultural competence assessment profile*. Retrieved from: www.hrsa.gov/culturalcompetence/healthdlvr.pdf

The providers' guide to quality and culture Retrieved from: http://erc.msh.org/mainpage.cfm?file=1.0.htm&module=provider&language=English American Academy of Family Physicians

Cultural proficiency resources. Retrieved from: www.aafp.org/online/en/home/clinical/publichealth/culturalprof.html American Academy of Pediatrics

Cultural competency (starter kit for community preceptors). Retrieved from: http://practice.aap.org/content.aspx?aID=1757

Motivational interviewing. Retrieved from: http://www.motivation alinterview.org/

Multicultural health in public health practice. Retrieved from: http://www.njphtc.org/

Practicing cross-cultural communication: Ongoing, free online training course of the New York/ New Jersey Public Health Training Center. Retrieved from: http://www.phtc-online.org/learning/pages/ catalog/cc/

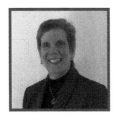 **Jeanette Panchula** has been a La Leche League Leader since 1975, an IBCLC since 1985, and most recently worked as a Senior Public Health Nurse in California. She works part-time as a consultant for the Maternal, Child, and Adolescent Health Divisions of the state of California and Solano County. She enjoys speaking/teaching about breastfeeding and communication to hospital staff and peer counselors alike.

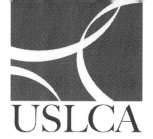

Working with Families of Different Cultures, Part II

Families of Different Cultures

Jeanette Panchula BSW, RN, PHN, IBCLC, RLC[1]

Keywords: Breastfeeding, cultural competence, communication skills

Working with families from different cultures requires self-awareness, the desire to understand the goals of our clients, and the ability to collaborate with them to achieve the outcome they are seeking. Primarily this is achieved through asking open-ended questions, listening not just to the words, but the feelings that are being communicated, sharing with her that what she has stated is understood, and then helping her identify an option that will work for her, her baby, and her family. Using this method maintains respect for the client's beliefs and culture, and increases the likelihood of a successful outcome—and possibly creating a new breastfeeding expert and advocate in the process.

---

1   jeanette.panchula@sbcglobal.net

As an IBCLC, it is essential that we not only have knowledge of the information that will help a mother breastfeed. We also have to know how to impart that knowledge. Below are some suggestions I've compiled from my backgrounds in Social Work, La Leche League Leadership, and local, state, and national WIC projects. I have helped mothers breastfeed in Puerto Rico, and five different U.S. states.

The Code of Professional Conduct for IBCLCs states:

> 1.2 Provide care to meet clients' individual needs that is culturally appropriate and informed by the best available evidence.

In order to accomplish this, we must take responsibility to understand the families we serve. We can increase our knowledge just as we do for other aspects of our work as IBCLCs.

If you do a web search of *cultural competence*, you will find lists of courses available from many sources. Often these courses and books provide lists of what *they* believe. Although interesting and possibly a way to help the IBCLC know what questions to ask, these can also lead us to assume that *we know* what *this mother* believes; a concept that is, in my opinion, as useless as knowing what *Americans* or *Southerners* believe.

The publication of an essay about *Cultural Humility* better reflects the need to develop a lifelong skill, and the ability to learn and discern appropriate care for our clients, as described in the website by California Health Advocates: Are you practicing cultural humility? The key to success in cultural competence. www.cahealthadvocates.org/news/disparities/2007/are-you.html

Dr. Melanie Tervalon and Jann Murray-Garcia describe cultural humility as a lifelong process of self-reflection and self-critique. The starting point for such an approach is not an examination of the client's belief system, but rather having health care/service providers give careful consideration to their assumptions and beliefs that are embedded in their own understandings and goals of their encounters with clients.

An IBCLC can increase his/her skill by:

» Reading books, such as *Women's Ways of Knowing* (Belenky et al., 1997), or this article by Monica Roosa Ordway (2008). http://jhl.sagepub.com/content/24/2/135.full.pdf+html

» Attending webinars such as:

   » *Promoting breastfeeding in minority communities and in the workplace.* http://www.albany.edu/sph/cphce/bfgr/bfgr04.htm

   » *Communicate to make a difference series: exploring cross cultural communication.* New York/New Jersey Public Health Training Center http://www.empirestatephtc.org/learning/pages/catalog/cc/

But most of all work towards increasing our knowledge through a variety of experiences. I encourage all IBCLCs who work in hospitals or private clinics to connect with professionals in public health, especially public-health nursing. Making home visits, and seeing what mothers will be facing when they go home, is one of the best ways to develop a better understanding of the *landscape* of our clients, including their culture.

Similar to when we lack knowledge about how to deal with mothers with different physical characteristics or situations from our own (e.g., larger breasts, twins), we must increase our ability to communicate with mothers with experiences we may not have had (e.g., poverty, racism).

IBCLCs spend a lot of time and effort preparing for the exam, and continue to take courses to maintain their certification. I believe, that like CPR and ethics, communication skills should also be a requirement for re-certifications. Often we *forget* what steps to follow when communicating with our clients. Of course, there is no *one way*. Below are some points I believe will help. Without developing the skills to communicate with our clients, there is much less likelihood that we will have met our client's needs, leading to frustration for both the IBCLC and the mother.

Self-Awareness

My first degree was Social Work. The training offered was related to using our own personalities to help improve communication with our clients. This required an awareness not only of our clients' needs, but also of ourselves. It is essential that we be aware of our own preconceived notions. This is the first step in working with our clients/patients. What if we are in a situation where we cannot avoid working with mothers who make us feel uncomfortable? We need to acknowledge to ourselves that this is the case, in order to avoid placing the burden of communication on our clients.

» We need to be very attuned to both their body language and tone of voice, and our own.

» **An example:** Perhaps we find teens annoying know-it-alls, difficult to communicate with, and unwilling to listen. What can we do?

» Be aware of this attitude.

» Identify others who enjoy working with teens and provide them with the knowledge of how to support these young, breastfeeding moms.

» If there is no one else, we must be very aware of our communication, especially non-verbal. Below will be some steps that will help.

You may wonder why I chose to use *teens* as an example in this article about *Working with mothers of different cultures?* I did this quite purposefully. I have found that when we consider *teens* a different culture, rather than as *unfinished adults* who *have no business being mothers*, and address them with similar respect as we would a mother from Bangladesh or Cuba or Laos, we are more successful in developing rapport, identifying their barriers, and developing a plan that will work in THEIR culture/landscapes.

Avoid Prescribing

Once we have become self-aware, we can more easily address the needs of our client. However, we need to have a *barrier to our lips* when we first meet with a mother.

We need to avoid walking in with *this is what you need to do* or *I understand you're having* _____*and it's best if you* _____.

> » ... even when we were given a written chart with clear documentation of what is troubling this mother ...

> » ... even when we talked to her on the telephone and she told us what she needed ...

> » ... even when a fellow IBCLC has described clearly what issues are ...

Some basic steps highlighted below can help us discover a mother's issues and solutions. (In WIC it is called the Three Steps. In other programs, there are more.)

As experts, we often move into a *fixing* mode, and then are frustrated when the mother *doesn't do it*. Mothers need to know, in their deepest self, that you have *heard* them: that you are not just giving them information and answers based on what *you* believe, but on what *they* are experiencing.

Clarify the Information

We must know what *this* mother is reporting, in her own words. Yes, it seems like a *waste of time*. But we accomplish two very important goals.

1. A mother will get to know us and develop a sense of being heard and understood. Thus, we avoid the trap of assuming we know what is truly her concern.

2. We will hear symptoms in *her* words rather than interpretations by others, which can often lead to a different plan, and save us a great deal of time in the long run.

We accomplish this through the use of what we have learned through many different venues and professional courses: Ask open-ended questions.

If we ask: *Does it hurt?* We get a *yes* or *no* answer. In contrast, if we ask: *What does it feel like?*, or *What was the last feeding like?*, or *Can you describe your day to me?*, we get a much richer description, which often leads to additional questions.

Continue to Clarify

After we have some ideas of what is going on, describe back what you heard and make sure you heard it correctly, or that you did not misinterpret a term. This is especially important. Terms and language mean different words to different cultural groups. For example, you may assume you understand what *Hispanics* mean. But if you are talking to a Puerto Rican, *ahorita* means *in the near future.* To a Mexican mom, it means *right now.* This misunderstanding can cause big problems in terms of scheduling a visit, starting a treatment, or arranging for a referral.

An African American mother may say to you that her baby is *greedy.* Does that mean the baby is too demanding? Or does it mean that her baby is strong, knows what he wants, and goes for it?

Another important clarifying question: What have you tried?

Asking this shows respect for the mother. She must have tried *something* if her baby was crying, or too sleepy, or not latching on correctly. Listening to the mother can often reduce the frustration often felt by IBCLCs who say, *she refuses to try anything I suggest!* Some may say: Asking all these questions will take *tooo long!*

In my experience, without asking questions and getting a full picture, a lot of time is wasted, teaching what has already been tried, or worse: providing education on what is not the real problem. For example, a mother calls and says her nipples are sore. Until we ask questions about the age of the baby, when this started, what happens and when, what it looks like, we could be giving information about positioning when the issue is that the baby bit her.

Reflect Feelings and Validate

After asking questions and clarifying information, many IBCLCs launch into the *teaching* mode:

> » *What you need to do is: ...* Or

> » *Let's get the baby going ...* Or

> » *I need to refer you to ...*

However, if a mother does not sense that we understand what they have been through, she often will just repeat a description of her problem, at times almost verbatim, again. They seem to give us a *broken record* report, stating over and over their issues.

For example:

> » *No one listened.*

> » *They didn't help me.*

> » *The labor was horrible.*

> » *When the baby latches on it, feels like crushed glass.*

I've found that mothers need to know we *heard* them and understand what they feel, and what has upset them.

It is hard at times to remember to take this step. We want to get going on the *fixing* stage. However, when working with mothers of our own, or of different cultures, and especially with mothers for whom English is not the first language, it is one of the best ways to establish a feeling of trust and understanding. Choose words you are comfortable with, and be specific so the mother knows you care.

> » *It sounds like you've been very frustrated with different solutions given to you.*

> » *How frightened you must have felt when you learned your baby was losing weight.*

> » *You're feeling guilty about not wanting to breastfeed. But it hurts too much!*

It is important to use different and specific feeling words. We don't have to fear getting it *wrong;* mothers will usually correct us if we didn't get it *right* (e.g., *No, I'm not frightened. I'm ANGRY.*). Doing this gives us time to really listen, think the solution through for this breastfeeding dyad, rather than running headlong into the *education mode.* In my experience, when mothers sense that we DO understand and are *with* them in their feelings, they more easily move on to the next step: addressing their issues and problem-solving *with* us.

Targeted Education

Whatever culture or language, mothers of young babies and mothers under stress are not ready to hear a large number of instructions. Our education must be targeted to the problem at hand, and what mother is ready to hear. This can be difficult for us. We want her to know ... so much more.

> » What her baby needs at 1 day, at 7 days, at 2 months, etc.

» Babies need to be *babied*.

» This period of total dependence is really very short in the *big picture*.

» Breastfeeding will make a huge difference in their relationship with their babies, and their babies' health.

The reality is the mom is not ready to hear so many messages. We must concentrate on her question, her priorities, and her concerns. We need to identify what she feels she needs to know, answer her questions by giving her various options—even those you would rather she not take, and then be open to listening to her decision.[1]

For example, a mother has decided her nipples hurt too much, even though she was able to latch the baby to the breast with little pain while you were there, she wants to pump. This is not the time to disagree with her. It is the time to let her know you respect her decision, and will be available to address other options when she is ready. Provide email, telephone, and web contact information that she can use to access you or someone who can translate if she cannot communicate directly with you.

Following Up

Maintaining contact with mothers of different cultures and languages can be difficult. Whenever possible follow-up the visit with a text or an email (even mothers who are poor now have access to the Internet) with links to information in their language to send a follow-up email. Some sources are:

> » **La Leche League International**
>   www.lalecheleague.org
>
> » **Medline**
>   www.nlm.nih.gov/medlineplus/languages/ breastfeeding.html
>
> » **The Baby Friendly Initiative, UK**
>   http://www.unicef.org.uk/BabyFriendly/ Resources/Resources-in-other-languages/

Having used the steps above often leads to a continuing relationship with mothers, giving us opportunities to add to our own knowledge of their culture and beliefs. This will also allow us to develop the skills of someone who will someday be able to provide information and support to her friends and neighbors—in their own language.

In my experience, this is one of the most rewarding aspects of my job as an IBCLC: meeting a mother who is breastfeeding and learning from her that a mother I helped years ago, helped her. I can see a network of knowledgeable and multicultural experts growing, as these mothers become Peer Counselors and IBCLCs!

References

Airhihenbuwa, C.O. (1995). *Health and culture-beyond the western paradigm.* Thousand Oaks, CA: Sage Publications.

Beasley, A. (1991). Breastfeeding studies: Culture, biomedicine, and methodology. *Journal of Human Lactation: 7; 7.*

Belenky, M.F. et al. (1997). *Women's ways of knowing: The development of self, voice, and mind.* New York City, Basic Books

Bodo, K., & Gibson, N. (1999). Childbirth customs in Orthodox Jewish traditions. *Canadian Family Physician. 45,* 682–686. Retrieved from: http://www.ncbi.nlm.nih.gov/pmc/articles/PMC2328400/?page=1

Chiu, S.H., Anderson, G.C., & Burkhammer, M.D. (2008). Skin-toskin contact for culturally diverse women having reastfeeding difficulties during the early postpartum. *Breastfeeding Medicine, 3*(4), 231–237

Good Mojab, C. (2000). The cultural art of breastfeeding. *Leaven, 36*(5), 87–91.

Hunt, L.M. (2001). *Beyond cultural competence applying humility to clinical settings. Up front.* Retrieved from: http://www.parkridgecenter.org/Page1882.html

Kiselica, M. S. (1995). *Multicultural counseling with teenage fathers.* Thousand Oaks, CA: Sage Publications.

Lauwers. J., & Swisher, A. (2005). *Counseling the nursing mother,* 4th ed. Sudbury, MA: Jones and Bartlett.

Lu, M.C., & Halfon, M. (2003). Racial and ethnic disparities in birth outcomes: A life-course perspective. *Maternal and Child Health Journal, 7*(1), 13–30

Mohrbacker, N. (2010). *Breastfeeding answers made simple.* Amarillo, TX: Hale Publishing.

Ordway, M.R. (2008). Synthesizing breastfeeding research: A commentary on the use of *Women's ways of knowing. Journal of Human Lactation, 24,* 135-138.

Riordan, J., (2010). *Breastfeeding and human lactation, 5th Ed..* Sudbury, MA: Jones and Bartlett.

Scott, J.A., & Mostyn, T. (2003). Women's experiences of breastfeeding in a bottle-feeding culture. *Journal of Human Lactation, 19,* 270.

Tervalon, M., & Murray-Garcia, J. (1998). Cultural humility versus cultural competence: A critical distinction in defining physician training outcomes in multicultural education. *Journal of Health Care for the Poor and Underserved, 9*(2), 117.

Thulier, D. (2009). Breastfeeding in America: A history of influencing factors. *Journal of Human Lactation, 25,* 85.

Zimmerman, G.L., Olsen, C.G., & Bosworth, M.F. (2000). *A "Stages of Change" approach to helping patients change behavior.* American Family Physician. Retrieved from: http://www.aafp. org/afp/20000301/1409.htm

Clinical Lactation, 2012, Vol. 3-1, 16-20

CAUTION

If there is fear for the baby's health, such as when a mother demands that she MUST exclusively breastfeed, we must be aware of our obligations. If, despite attempts to establish rapport and communicate with her effectively, there is still concern that her choice may put her baby at risk, it is essential that we communicate our concerns with the baby's health care provider. (Code of Professional Conduct for IBCLCs; 4.2 http://iblce.org/ wp-content/uploads/2013/08/code-of-professional-conduct.pdf)

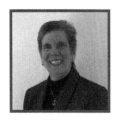 **Jeanette Panchula** has been a La Leche League Leader since 1975, an IBCLC since 1985, and most recently worked as a Senior Public Health Nurse in California. She works part-time as a consultant for the Maternal, Child, and Adolescent Health Divisions of the state of California and Solano County. She enjoys speaking/teaching about breastfeeding and communication to hospital staff and peer counselors alike.

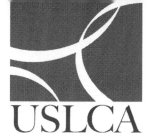

American Indian Breastfeeding Folklore from the Eastern Shoshone and Northern Arapaho Tribes

Diane Powers, BA, IBCLC, RLC
Vicki Bodley Tapia, BS, IBCLC, RLC

Keywords: American Indian, breastfeeding oral history, milk fever, induced lactation

Over the years, much of the folklore of breastfeeding has been lost because women did not write history, they told stories. This article shares breastfeeding lore from stories told to the authors by American Indian women from the Eastern Shoshone and Northern Arapaho tribes on the Wind River Reservation near Lander, Wyoming. These women related stories describing treatment for milk fever (mastitis), the White man's influence on mother/baby separation and its outcome, elderly women inducing lactation, breastfeeding and birth control, and how women

dressed for ease of breastfeeding in former times. It is
with appreciation for other cultures that we add this
information from American Indians to the archives
of breastfeeding history.

Would you feel comfortable joining the elders of the tribe native
to our area, in a circle-of-sharing during the noon-time break?
This unusual request was made to us during the morning
break on the second day of a two-day breastfeeding
conference we were presenting at a hospital in southern
Wyoming on the Wind River Reservation. We realized
this offer to join the circle was a rare opportunity for us, as
well as a sign of respect seldom offered to White women.
We did not hesitate to answer. *Yes, of course.*

Nearly 40 people filled the hospital conference room
that day in Lander, Wyoming. We hadn't noticed any
American Indians in the audience, but by the time twelve
o'clock arrived, the ethnicity in the room had shifted
noticeably. The tables set up classroom style for the morning
session were pushed to the outer edges of the room and a
circle of chairs materialized in the center of the room. As
the elders of the tribe began the session, they made a point
to invite everyone in the room to join them in the circle.
To our surprise, the Caucasian group standing with their
backs to the wall and the tables in front of them remained
motionless. Only the two of us walked into the center of the
room and found a seat in the circle.

The American Indian women began to speak. Using
their traditional oral history, these women shared stories

of breastfeeding in their culture. We both quickly sensed the reason they had requested our presence in their midst. It was apparent these women wanted their oral history about breastfeeding heard. We suspect they hoped their oral history might reach ears willing to transcribe their experiences into written history.

These determined women wanted us to hear how they were taught to treat such maladies as mastitis. They wanted us to understand how modern White men, in the name of progress, had thoughtlessly interrupted the special bond between mother and baby. They wanted us to visualize the dresses women wore which were designed so breastfeeding was easy as they went about their daily chores. The emotions of these women as they told us their stories reflected a combination of pragmatism, pride, and indignation.

Mastitis and Plugged Ducts

Milk fever is an antiquated term for our present day word, mastitis. Prior to antibiotics, women sometimes died from *milk fever.* It was an infection not to be taken lightly. American Indian women were aware that this illness could be deadly and needed to be treated promptly. One of the women looked at us and remarked, *Do you know what American Indian women did when they had mastitis?* We both shook our heads *no.*

...In the time before electricity and breast pumps, if a mother had mastitis, someone found a newborn puppy to put to the woman's breast to suckle. We knew that a puppy's suck was much more powerful than that of a human baby. Because of the importance of draining as much milk as possible from the infected breast, the puppy's strong suck helped the mother recover. Unfortunately for the puppy, American Indian tradition required that the puppy be blinded before suckling at the woman's breast. In an attempt to repay the puppy for losing its eyesight, and to recognize his importance in the healing process, he was then considered part of the family and raised as a blood brother or sister to the baby.

One woman went on to tell us, *Plugged ducts were treated with a slab of fat, from a bear or bison, warmed over the fire and then placed on the red, painful area on the breast.*

Separating Mothers and Babies: The White Man's Influence

One of the women in the circle shared with sadness in her voice:

My mother-in-law breastfed two of my four children on an ongoing basis because of my need to work to support my family.

Her position with the Indian Health Service required that she be transplanted from southern Wyoming to Washington D.C. for weeks at a time when her first and second children were babies. The grandmother was left with the mother's frozen breast milk, but when that was depleted, the grandmother put the baby to the breast and gradually induced lactation.

Culturally, there was then pressure for the mother to *give* these children to the grandmother because breast-feeding was such an important spiritual tie between individuals in their culture. The end result was that two children, both breastfed by the grandmother, lived with the grandmother, and the other two stayed with their mother. It was now 20 years after the fact, but there was no missing the disappointment, wistfulness, and pain in this woman's voice as she told us her story.

Induced Lactation

As we sat in the circle that day, stories were told about grandmothers who induced lactation in order to breastfeed their grandchildren when the mothers disappeared. Worldwide, it has historically been reported that there are women who have induced lactation when necessity called, even though it might have been months or years since they last breastfed (Brewster, 1979; Lawrence & Lawrence, 2005; Riordan & Auerbach, 2005). As we listened, another story was remembered.

> … Very early one morning, two elderly American Indian women were foraging in the town dump. These women lived alone in a teepee as their men had died. They were expected to find their own food. Going through the garbage, they were

startled to find a newborn baby lying on top of the pile. The moisture of this yet wet newborn rose up in steam from the coolness of the morning air. The infant had blonde hair. As best we can piece together, the year was 1904.

As if the peace pipe had passed in the circle, another woman picked up the story line.

...Unable to leave the baby there to die, these nearly starving, older women took him back to their camp. He survived because both women put him to the breast, and even though it had been many years since they had breastfed, they brought their milk back and then raised him as their own. Tribal oral history reports that he grew up with the tribe and lived with them until adulthood, when he left.

Breastfeeding and Birth Control

Breastfeeding a child for 4 or 5 years was reported as not uncommon. In this way, breastfeeding was used as a means of birth control. When the mother was ready to wean, the child was sent to a sister's or close relative's home for four or five days.

American Indian women were taught if they became pregnant while breastfeeding, they must wean so the fetus would receive enough nourishment. After learning of her daughter's pregnancy, one grandmother was said to have chided her grandson, *You have to get off the breast; don't be a cannibal.*

Fashion for Breastfeeding

Advice given by the wise women of the tribe to first-time mothers included the admonition, *wear a vest when breast-feeding to help cover wet spots caused by leaking milk.* They also wore long dresses with slits in the dress to facilitate the ease of breastfeeding.

As we listened to these stories told by the Native women, we were at times amazed and continually captivated by what they shared. Over the years, much of the folklore of breastfeeding has been lost because women did not write history, they told stories. It is with appreciation for other cultures that we add this information from American Indians to the archives of breastfeeding history.

Clinical Lactation, 2011, Vol. 2-4, 30-31

References

Brewster, D.A. (1979). *You can breastfeed your baby.* Emmaus, PA: Rodale Press.

Lawrence, R.A., & Lawrence, R.M. (2005). *Breastfeeding: A guide for the medical profession* (6th ed.). Philadelphia: Elsevier Mosby Press.

Riordan, J., & Auerbach, K. (2005). *Breastfeeding and human lactation* (3rd ed.). Sudbury, MA: Jones & Bartlett Publishers.

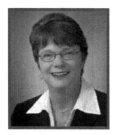

Diane Powers, BA, IBCLC, RLC, is a lactation consultant and former La Leche League leader. For the past 23 years, she has worked with approximately 700 new mother/baby pairs per year, both in-patient and outpatient. She has completed two research projects and had numerous articles published. She lectures nationally and internationally.

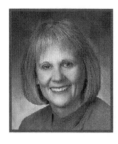

Vicki Bodley Tapia, B.S., IBCLC, RLC, is a former La Leche League Leader, and has been in private practice as a lactation consultant since 1987, published numerous articles, and lectures both nationally and internationally. She is the author of *Somebody Stole My Iron: A Family Memoir of Dementia* from Praeclarus Press.

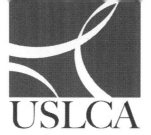

Breastfeeding and Racial/Ethnic Disparities in Infant Mortality

Celebrating Successes and Overcoming Barriers

Kathleen Kendall-Tackett, PhD, IBCLC, RLC, FAPA[1]

Keywords: Breastfeeding, racial/ethnic health disparities, infant mortality, bedsharing

Many exciting changes occurred in 2013 in the breast-feeding world. One of the best changes was the increase in breastfeeding rates in the African American community. In 2013, the Centers for Disease Control and Prevention (CDC) indicated that increased breastfeeding in African American women narrowed the gap in infant mortality rates (http://www.cdc.gov/mmwr/preview/mmwrhtml/mm6205a1.htm#tab).

---

1   kkendallt@gmail.com

As the CDC noted:

> From 2000 to 2008, breastfeeding initiation increased ... from 47.4% to 58.9% among Blacks. Breastfeeding duration at 6 months increased from ... 16.9% to 30.1% among Blacks. Breastfeeding duration at 12 months increased from ... 6.3% to 12.5% among Blacks.

Much of this wonderful increase in breastfeeding rates among African Americans is the result of efforts within that community.

In 2013, we saw the first Black Breastfeeding Week become part of World Breastfeeding Week in the U.S. Programs, such as A More Excellent Way (http://www.mewpeers.org/), Reaching Our Sisters Everywhere (ROSE; http://www.breastfeedingrose.org/main-page/), and Free to Breastfeed (http://freetobreastfeed.com/), offer peer counselor programs for African American women.

We can celebrate these successes. But there is still more to do. Although the rates of infant mortality have dropped, African American babies are still twice as likely to die compared to White babies. In addition, although rates of breastfeeding have increased among African Americans, they are still lower than they are for other ethnic groups (http://www.cdc.gov/mmwr/preview/mmwrhtml/mm6205a1.htm#tab).

> For each of the 2000–2008 birth years, breast-feeding initiation and duration prevalences were significantly lower among Black infants compared

with White and Hispanic infants. However, the gap between Black and White breastfeeding initiation narrowed from 24.4 percentage points in 2000 to 16.3 percentage points in 2008.

Barriers to Overcome

To continue this wonderful upward trend in breastfeeding rates, we need to acknowledge possible barriers to breast-feeding among African American women.

Here are a couple of barriers I've observed. They are not the only ones. But they are ones I've consistently encountered. Addressing these will not be a quick fix, but these barriers can be overcome if we recognize them and take appropriate action.

1. **Pathways for IBCLCs of Color.** In their book, *Birth Ambassadors*, Christine Morton and Elayne Clift highlight a problem in the doula world that also has relevance for the lactation world: most doulas (and International Board Certified Lactation Consultants [IBCLCs]) are White, middle-class women. And there is a very practical reason for this. This is generally the only demographic of women that can afford to become doulas (or IBCLCs). The low pay, or lack of job opportunities for IBCLCs who are not also nurses, means that there are limited opportunities for women without other sources of income to be in this profession. Also, as we limit tracks for peer counselors to become IBCLCs, we limit the

opportunities for women of color to join our field. I recently met a young African American woman who told me that she would love to become an IBCLC, but couldn't get the contact hours needed to sit for the exam. That's a shame. (I did refer her to someone I knew could help.)

2. We need to have some dialogue about how we can bring along the next generation of IBCLCs. We need to recognize the structural barriers that make it difficult for young women of color to enter our field. And these discussions can start with you. Sherry Payne, in her recent webinar, *Welcoming African American Women into Your Practice* , recommends that professionals who work in communities of color find their replacement from the communities they serve. Even if you only mentor one woman of color to become an IBCLC, you can have a tremendous impact in your community. If we all do the same, we can change the face of our field.

3. **Bedsharing and Breastfeeding.** This is an issue that I expect will become more heated over the next couple of years. But it is a reality. As we encourage more women to breastfeed, a higher percentage of them will bedshare. As recent studies have repeatedly found, bedsharing increases breastfeeding duration. This is particularly true for exclusive breastfeeding (Ball, 2007; Lahr, Rosenberg, & Lapidus, 2007; Middlemiss & Kendall-Tackett, 2014).

Bedsharing is a particular concern when we are talking about breastfeeding in the African American community (Lahr et al., 2007; Middlemiss & Kendall-Tackett, 2014). Of all ethnic groups studied, bedsharing is most common in African Americans. It is unrealistic to think that we are going to simultaneously increase breastfeeding rates while decreasing bedsharing rates in this community. The likely scenario is that breastfeeding would falter. It's interesting that another recent CDC report, *Public Health Approaches to Reducing U.S. Infant Mortality*, talks quite a bit about safe-sleep messaging, with barely a mention of breastfeeding in decreasing infant mortality (http://www.cdc. gov/mmwr/preview/mmwrhtml/mm6231a3.htm). A more constructive approach might be to talk about being safe while bedsharing. But as long as the message is simply *never bedshare*, there is likely to be little progress, and it could potentially become a barrier to breastfeeding.

Reason to Hope

Even with these barriers, and others I haven't listed, Baby-Friendly Hospitals are having a positive effect. When hospitals have Baby-Friendly policies in place, racial disparities in breastfeeding rates seem to disappear. For example, a study of 32 U.S. Baby-Friendly Hospitals revealed breastfeeding initiation rates of 83.8%, compared to the (then) national average of 69.5%. In-hospital exclusive breastfeeding rates were 78.4%, compared with a national rate of 46.3%. *Rates were similar even for hospitals with high proportions of Black or low-income patients* (Merewood, Mehta, Chamberlain, Phillipp, & Bauchner, 2005). This is a very hopeful sign, especially as more hospitals in the U.S. go Baby-Friendly. But we need to make sure that we follow Step 10, and that mothers have great support in their communities once they leave the hospital.

In summary, we have made significant strides in reducing the high rates of infant mortality in the U.S., particularly among African Americans. I am encouraged by the large interest in this topic, and the number of different groups working toward this goal. Keep up the good work. I think we are reaching critical mass.

Clinical Lactation, 2012, Vol. 3-1, 26-29

References

Ball, H. L. (2007). Night-time infant care: Cultural practice, evolution, and infant development. In P. Laimputtong (Ed.), *Childreading and infant care issues* (pp. 1–15). Hauppauge, NY: Nova Science Publishers.

Lahr, M. B., Rosenberg, K. D., & Lapidus, J. A. (2007). Maternal-infant bedsharing: Risk factors for bedsharing in a population-based survey of new mothers and implications for SIDS risk reduction. *Maternal Child Health Journal, 11,* 277–286.

Merewood, A., Mehta, S. D., Chamberlain, L. B., Phillipp, B. L., & Bauchner, H. (2005). Breastfeeding rates in U.S. Baby-Friendly hospitals: Results of a national survey. *Pediatrics, 116*(3), 628–634.

Middlemiss, W., & Kendall-Tackett, K. A. (Eds.). (2014). *The science of mother-infant sleep: Current findings on bedsharing, breastfeeding, sleep training, and normal infant sleep.* Amarillo, TX: Praeclarus Press.

Helpful Links

Black Mothers' Breastfeeding Summit,
http://youtube/b8MXkKkO1a4

Teach Me to Breastfeed Rap,
http://www.youtube.com/watch?v=ax85hE3_2uE

Interview With Sherry Payne on Fighting Breastfeeding Disparities With Support, http://kcur.org/post/kc-group-fights-breast-feedingdisparities-education-support

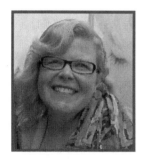

Kathleen Kendall-Tackett, PhD, IBCLC, RLC, FAPA, is a health psychologist and an International Board Certified Lactation Consultant. She is the owner and editor-in-chief of Praeclarus Press, a small press specializing in women's health. Dr. Kendall-Tackett is a fellow of the American Psychological Association in both the Divisions of Health and Trauma Psychology and clinical associate professor of Pediatrics at Texas Tech University School of Medicine in Amarillo, Texas.

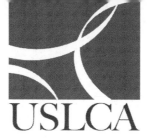

Addressing Racial and Ethnic Health Disparities in Infant Mortality

Additional Barriers to Care

Kathleen Kendall-Tackett, PhD, IBCLC, RLC, FAPA[1]

Keywords: Infant mortality, racial/ethnic health disparities, obesity

In 2013, the Centers for Disease Control and Prevention reported that the infant mortality rate among African Americans had dropped (http://www.cdc.gov/mmwr/preview/mmwrhtml/mm6205a1.htm#tab). It was an amazing and hopeful finding. In addition, they attributed this drop to breastfeeding. It was Christmas in July! We should take a moment to celebrate this tremendous success and commend the community organizations that helped make it happen. Your work has been amazing.

1   kkendallt@gmail.com

Of course, there is still much to do and several more issues we need to address before racial/ethnic disparities in infant mortality can be eliminated. A partial list follows.

Trauma History

Psychological trauma is not something we usually think about as being related to breastfeeding. But it can be a barrier. And there are racial/ethnic group differences in percentages of women who've experienced trauma. Black women are significantly more likely to report a history of trauma than White women.

For example, in a national survey of 1,581 pregnant women, Black women had more lifetime posttraumatic stress disorder (PTSD) and trauma exposure than White women. When looking at current prevalence of PTSD, Black women were four times more likely to have PTSD compared with other women in the sample. This rate did not vary by socioeconomic status and it was explained by greater trauma exposure (Seng, Kohn-Wood, McPherson, & Sperlich, 2011).

Women's history of trauma is difficult for them. It also has some serious implications for the health of their babies. PTSD in pregnancy can lead to several serious complications including low birthweight and shorter gestation. For example, in one study of 839 pregnant women, women with PTSD in pregnancy had babies that weighed an average of 283 g less than babies of women without PTSD. PTSD was a stronger predictor of low birthweight for African

American babies than it was for other babies in the sample (Seng, Low, Sperlich, Ronis, & Liberzon, 2011).

Our data from the Survey of Mothers' Sleep and Fatigue indicated that breastfeeding can help women who have a trauma history. We examined the impact of previous sexual assault on women's postpartum experience. Our sample included 994 sexual assault survivors. As expected, women who had been sexually assaulted had more sleep problems, anxiety, depression, anger, and irritability. But when we added feeding method to the analyses, we found that exclusive breastfeeding actually attenuated the effects of the trauma on all of these variables (Kendall-Tackett, Cong, & Hale, 2013). With so many mothers having a history of trauma, these findings are good news. But we need to be realistic in recognizing that a trauma history can be a barrier to breastfeeding, even though it can lessen the impact of trauma.

PTSD is often related to a history of interpersonal violence. It can also be caused by the woman's birth experience. Here, too, African American women are more vulnerable. In the Childbirth Connection's Listening to Mothers II survey, 9% of the total sample met full criteria for PTSD following traumatic childbirth experiences, and 18% of the total sample had posttraumatic stress symptoms. When these numbers were broken out by ethnicity, 26% of Black women had posttraumatic stress symptoms following their births, compared to 18% for the full sample and 14% of Hispanic women (Beck, Gable, Sakala, & Declercq, 2011). This raises the question of why

Black women were more likely to have traumatic births. Perhaps part of the answer lies in how birth was handled for them. And that's related to the next issue.

Weight Bias

Our maternity care system treats women with higher body mass indexes (BMIs) in some very discriminatory ways, often shunting them off into high-risk maternity care whether they need it or not; these decisions are simply made based on women's weight—with or without other health risks.

This practice differentially impacts Black women because there are significantly higher percentages of women of color who fall into *overweight* and *obese* categories, as you can see in Figure 1.

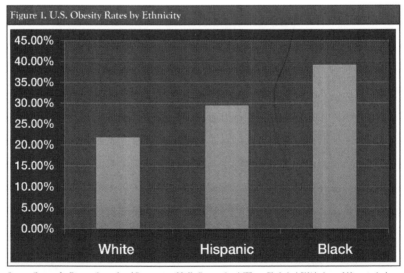

Figure 1. U.S. Obesity Rates by Ethnicity

Source: Centers for Disease Control and Prevention. (2010). *Compared with Whites, Blacks had 51% higher and Hispanics had 21% higher obesity rates*. Retrieved from http://www.cdc.gov/Features/dsObesityAdults

Women with higher BMIs are more likely to experience high-intervention births, including elective procedures. For example, in a meta-analysis of 11 studies, cesarean sections were 1.5 times more likely in women with BMIs > 26 and 2.25 times more likely in women with BMIs > 30 (Poobalan, Aucott, Gurung, Smith, & Bhattacharya, 2009). Someone reading this finding might assume that high BMIs made labor difficult and therefore these mothers ended up with cesarean sections. That assumption would be only partially correct. Heavier women are also more likely to have *elective* cesareans than their thinner counterparts. In the Poobalan et al. (2009) study, obese women were almost twice as likely to have elective cesareans compared to women with lower BMIs. If women with higher BMIs are encouraged to have elective cesareans, there will be more Black women having cesareans. This demographic reality could account for the higher rate of birth trauma. and could also have a negative impact on breastfeeding.

Sleep

Several recent studies have found a link between experiences of everyday discrimination and sleep problems in ethnic minorities.

For example, in a study comparing Black and White adults, Blacks had shorter sleep duration and lower sleep efficiency. It took Blacks 25 minutes to fall asleep, compared to 16 minutes for Whites. Slow-wave sleep was similarly affected: 3.6% of total sleep was slow-wave compared to 6.8% for Whites (Mezick et al., 2008). Slow-wave sleep is the deeper stage of sleep. A smaller percentage is associated with more daytime fatigue and pain. This difference persisted even after controlling for socioeconomic status. Both of these sleep problems indicate chronic hyperarousal.

In another study of 97 Black and White adults, perceived unfair treatment for both groups was associated with poorer sleep quality, more daytime fatigue, shorter sleep duration, and a smaller proportion of rapid eye movement (REM). Overall, Blacks had lower sleep time and poorer sleep efficiency compared to Whites (Beatty et al., 2011).

These ethnic differences in sleep problems will likely be compounded when talking about sleep in new mothers. Fortunately, exclusive breastfeeding helps mothers to get more sleep (Kendall-Tackett, Cong, & Hale, 2011). But sleep may still continue to be an issue that impacts Black mothers' health and well-being, and may need to be separately addressed if breastfeeding is going to continue.

In summary, we have found that the causes of ethnic health disparities can be complex and daunting. Breast-feeding helps with many of these problems, but it can also be derailed if these other issues are not addressed. By protecting, promoting, and supporting breastfeeding, we can continue to decrease our infant mortality rate. But we need to recognize that health disparities do not lend themselves to quick fixes. Rather, interventions must take into account the whole of women's experiences to be effective.

References

Beatty, D. L., Hall, M. H., Kamarck, T. W., Buysse, D. J., Owens, J. F., Reis, S. E., ... Matthews, K. A. (2011). Unfair treatment is associated with poor sleep in African American and Caucasian adults: Pittsburgh Sleep-SCORE Project. *Health Psychology, 30*(3), 351–359.

Beck, C. T., Gable, R. K., Sakala, C., & Declercq, E. R. (2011). Posttraumatic stress disorder in new mothers: Results from a two-stage U.S. national survey. *Birth, 38*(3), 216–227.

Kendall-Tackett, K. A., Cong, Z., & Hale, T. W. (2011). The effect of feeding method on sleep duration, maternal well-being, and postpartum depression. *Clinical Lactation, 2*(2), 22–26.

Kendall-Tackett, K. A., Cong, Z., & Hale, T. W. (2013). Depression, sleep quality, and maternal well-being in postpartum women with a history of sexual assault: A comparison of breastfeeding, mixed-feeding, and formula-feeding mothers. *Breastfeeding Medicine, 8*(1), 16–22.

Mezick, E. J., Matthews, K. A., Hall, M., Strollo, P. J., Buysse, D. J., Kamarck, T. W., ... Reis, S. E. (2008). Influence of race and socioeconomic status on sleep: Pittsburgh Sleep-SCORE Project. *Psychosomatic Medicine, 70*, 410–416.

Poobalan, A. S., Aucott, L. S., Gurung, T., Smith, W. C. S., & Bhattacharya, S. (2009). Obesity as an independent risk factor for elective and emergency caesarean delivery in nulliparous women: Systematic review and meta-analysis of cohort studies. *Obesity Reviews, 10*, 28–35.

Seng, J. S., Kohn-Wood, L. P., McPherson, M. D., & Sperlich, M. A. (2011). Disparity in posttraumatic stress disorder diagnosis among African American pregnant women. *Archives of Women's Mental Health, 14*(4), 295–306.

Seng, J. S., Low, L. K., Sperlich, M. A., Ronis, D. L., & Liberzon, I. (2011). Posttraumatic stress disorder, child abuse history, birth weight, and gestational age: A prospective cohort study. *British Journal of Obstetrics & Gynecology, 118*(11), 1329–1339.

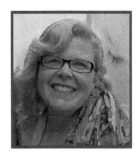 **Kathleen Kendall-Tackett, PhD, IBCLC, RLC, FAPA,** is a health psychologist, an International Board Certified Lactation Consultant, and the owner and editor-in-chief of Praeclarus Press, a small press specializing in women's health. Dr. Kendall-Tackett is editor-in-chief of *Clinical Lactation*, fellow of the American Psychological Association (APA) in Health and Trauma Psychology, past-president of the APA Division of Trauma Psychology, and editor-in-chief of *Psychological Trauma*.

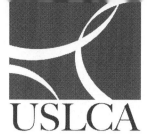

Trauma, Inflammation, and Racial/Ethnic Health Disparities

Kathleen Kendall-Tackett, PhD, IBCLC, RLC, FAPA

Keywords: Ethnic health disparities, preterm birth, trauma, sleep

According to the National Institutes of Health, health disparities refer to differences between groups of people. These differences can affect how frequently a disease affects a group, how many people get sick, or how often the disease causes death. Over the past 20 years, researchers, advocates, and public health officials have documented, and tried to address, the striking health disparities between racial/ethnic minority populations and Whites. The differences between Blacks and Whites are particularly striking and have been frequently documented in research studies. Some of these disparities include rates of infant mortality, obesity, cardiovascular disease, metabolic syndrome and diabetes, resulting in overall premature mortality.

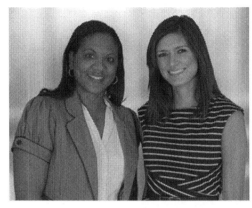

Health disparities refer to differences between groups of people. These differences can affect how frequently a disease affects a group, how many people get sick, or how often the disease causes death

National Institutes of Health (2014)

Disparities in Infant Mortality Rates

The rate of infant mortality is 5.5 per 1000 for Whites and 12.4 for Blacks. This rate actually reflects an improvement. Until last year, it was 13.8 per 1000. (The CDC credits the increase in breastfeeding rates among African Americans for this decrease.) This dismal statistic accounts for the fact that the U.S. is ranked 41st in the world in terms of infant mortality. Infant mortality is a key index of overall health of a country. Our rank puts us behind many developing countries.

Infant Death Rates per 1,000 Live Births

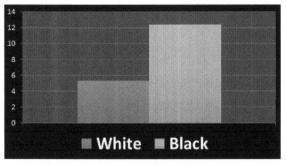

MMWR Feb 8 2013/ 62(5); 90

Much of the high mortality rate among Black infants is due to high rates of preterm birth. According to the World Health Organization, preterm birth is the number one cause of infant mortality. Here too there is a disparity.

Percentage of Preterm Births

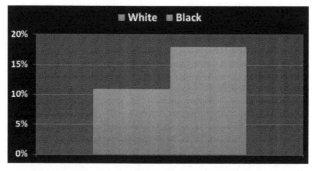

http://www.cdc.gov/nchs/data/nvsr/nvsr59/nvsr59_01.pdf

Racial/Ethnic Differences in Obesity Rates

Obesity rates also show striking ethnic-group differences, with African Americans having significantly higher rates than Whites.

U.S. Obesity Rates by Ethnicity

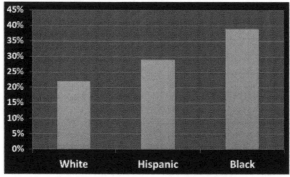

CDC, 2010, http://www.cdc.gov/Features/dsObesityAdults/

Interestingly, a similar pattern appears for indigenous people in Australia and Maori and Pacific Islanders in New Zealand.

Australian Obesity Rates for Women

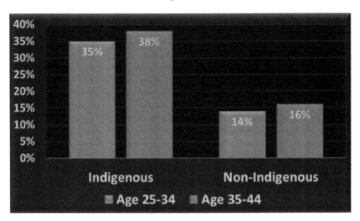

New Zealand Obesity Rates for Women

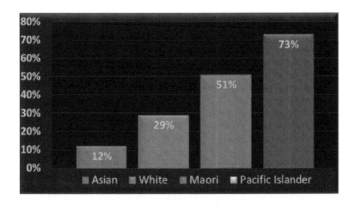

There is also a similar pattern based on socioeconomic status, with lower-income people having significantly higher rates.

U.S. Obesity Rates by Income

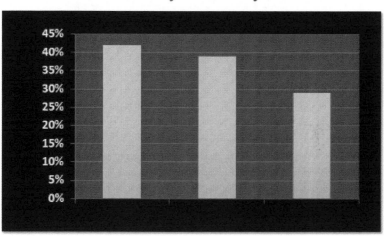

National Center on Health Statistics 2011

Diabetes and Heart Disease

We see similar patterns in rates of diabetes, metabolic syndrome, and heart disease, particularly for African Americans and American Indians. For example, the rate for diabetes in the U.S. is 7.6 per 1000 for Whites, 13.2 for non-Hispanic Blacks, and 15.6 for American Indians/ Alaska Natives (Centers for Disease Control and Prevention, 2014b). Not surprisingly, African American men tend to die at a younger age than men or women of other ethnic groups (Centers for Disease Control and Prevention, 2014a). (Hispanic women have the greatest longevity.)

What may surprise you is that these various manifestations of health disparity have the same underlying physiology. Inflammation, or more specifically, the upregulation of the inflammatory response system, underlies them all. To understand these inflammation effects, we need to draw from research in the field of psychoneuroimmunology. Trauma intersects with these physiological effects in some interesting ways, and enhances them (Kendall-Tackett, 2010b).

The Physiology of Stress

In a simplified form, we can think of the stress response as having three key components (Kendall-Tackett, 2010b).

The first is the catecholamine, or fight-or-flight response. In response to perceived threat, our bodies secrete three neurotransmitters: epinephrine, norepinephrine, and dopamine.

The second component of the stress response is the HPA axis. HPA stands for hypothalamic-pituitary-adrenal. This is a cascade response, meaning that in response to threat, the hypothalamus secretes the stress hormone CRH, which causes the pituitary to secrete the stress hormone ACTH, which causes the cortex of the adrenal gland to secrete the stress hormone cortisol.

The third component of the stress response is the immune response. In response to threat, the immune system increases inflammation by releasing proinflammatory cytokines, messenger molecules of the immune system. These molecules have two important functions: fighting infections and healing wounds. When under threat, the body prepares for possible attack—and injury—by being ready to heal wounds.

All components of the stress response are adaptive, meaning that they increase the likelihood of survival. This three-part stress response is meant to be acute: it turns on and it turns back off when the threat is over. The problem is that chronic stress, trauma, or even daily social rejection can keep this system activated, and that increases the likelihood of disease.

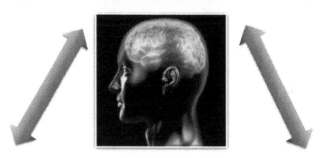

The Metabolic Syndrome

One other physiological state is necessary to describe, and that is the metabolic syndrome. The metabolic syndrome is the precursor syndrome to type-2 diabetes and is also a risk factor for heart disease (Haffner & Taegtmeyer, 2003). There are four key symptoms of the metabolic syndrome: insulin resistance, high LDL and VLDL cholesterol, high triglycerides, and visceral (abdominal) obesity. Metabolic syndrome, particularly insulin resistance, is related to increased inflammation and inflammation increases insulin resistance. Both are related to a chronically upregulated stress system.

Social Rejection and Inflammation: The Key to Understanding Health Disparities

In the introduction to the recent book, *Social Pain* (Jenson-Campbell & MacDonald, 2011), the authors describe how we are designed to be in relationship with each other. That being socially connected increases our chances of survival and that being part of a group provides resources, protection, and safety. When we perceive that we are not part of a group, we experience this rejection in the same part of our brains that process physical pain: the anterior cingulate cortex. Physiologically, humans experience social rejection as a threat to their physical survival (Dickerson, 2011; Eisenberger, 2011; Panksepp, 2011).

Microaggressions and Physical Health

Given that social rejection is perceived as a threat to survival, it's reasonable to hypothesize that it would increase inflammation. And it does. Health psychologists have documented that "perceived discrimination" (i.e., perceiving yourself as low in the social hierarchy) increases inflammation. In one study of 296 African Americans, Lewis et al. (2006) found that self-reported experiences of discrimination increased C-reactive protein (CRP; a common marker of chronic inflammation. It predicts risk of cardiovascular disease). Their measure included the following questions:

» You are treated with less courtesy than other people.

» You are treated with less respect than other people.

» You receive poorer service than other people at restaurants and stores.

» People act as if they think you are not smart.

In another study (McDade, Hawkley, & Cacioppo, 2006), perceived low social status was related to elevated C-reactive protein. This was a 3-year longitudinal study of 188 middle-aged and older adults. African Americans, women, and those with low education levels had the highest CRP. Another study (Hong, Nelesen, Krohn, Mills, & Dimsdale, 2006) found that perceived low social status was related to vascular inflammation, with elevated levels of the inflammatory molecules, ET-1 and sICAM. These effects were independent of hypertension status or ethnicity.

The effects of perceived discrimination can show up rather early. In a study of high school students (Goodman, McEwen, Huang, Dolan, & Adler, 2005), low parental education (a marker of socioeconomic status) predicted metabolic and cardiovascular risk factors including higher insulin levels, higher glucose, greater insulin resistance, higher HDL and lower LDL cholesterol, higher waist circumference, and higher BMI.

The Role of Sleep

Sleep is another factor that can be affected by everyday experiences of discrimination, and it too has a major impact on health (Kendall-Tackett, 2009b). For example, sleep problems can make you fat. In a meta-analysis of 36 studies (N=634,511 adults and children), short sleep duration (< 5 hours) was related to obesity worldwide (Cappuccio et al., 2008).

Sleep problems increase symptoms of metabolic syndrome and inflammation, thereby increasing the risk of diseases, such as heart disease and diabetes (Suarez & Goforth, 2010).

One study found that short sleep duration was related to metabolic syndrome in middle-aged adults (Hall et al., 2008). These symptoms included abdominal obesity, elevated fasting glucose, and high triglycerides. Suarez and Goforth (Suarez & Goforth, 2010) noted that even subclinical sleep disorders increase risk for cardiovascular disease, hypertension, type-2 diabetes, metabolic syndrome, and all-cause mortality. And even short periods of sleep deprivation (e.g., 1 or 2 days) can elevate cortisol and glucose levels, and increase insulin resistance (McEwen, 2003).

Ethnic Differences in Sleep

Given these health effects, it's interesting to note striking ethnic group differences in sleep. These could be the result of daily exposure to microaggressions or a result of trauma (or both). Either of these appear to upregulate the inflammatory response system. For example, a study of Black and White adults (N=187) found that Blacks had shorter sleep duration and lower sleep efficiency than whites (Mezick et al., 2008), taking longer to get to sleep and having a smaller percentage of slow-wave sleep.

Ethnic-Group Differences in Trauma

Trauma can also increase the risk of diseases, such as diabetes and heart disease, and it does it by increasing inflammation. For example, data from year 32 of the Dunedin Multidisciplinary Health and Development study, a birth-cohort study from Dunedin, New Zealand, revealed that those who experienced adverse childhood experiences (defined in this study as low SES, maltreatment, or social isolation) had higher rates of major depression, systemic inflammation, and having at least 3 metabolic risk markers (Danese et al., 2009).

Data from the Nurses' Health Study II, a study of more than 73,000 nurses, revealed that physical and sexual abuse in childhood or as a teen increased the risk of type-2 diabetes, even after adjusting for age, race, body type at age 5, parental education, and parental history of diabetes (Rich-Edwards et al., 2010).

Severity of abuse increased symptoms dramatically. There was a 50% increase in diabetes risk for those who experienced severe physical abuse and a 69% increase in risk in those who experienced repeated forced sex. Body Mass Index (BMI) was also influenced by past abuse. Physically and sexually abused girls had higher BMIs and the trajectories grew wider as the girls grew (i.e., they gained weight at a faster clip). This was particularly true for those who experienced repeated forced sex.

Unfortunately, there are ethnic group differences in experiences of trauma and the impact that it has. For example, a study of 177 Blacks and 822 Whites compiled a composite of early life adversities and 5 measures of inflammation. They found that early-life adversity predicted higher levels of inflammation for Blacks, but not Whites (Slopen et al., 2010).

Researchers from the Black Women's Health Study (N=33,298) found that early-life sexual and physical abuse was related to overall and central obesity (Boynton-Jarrett, Rosenberg, Palmer, Boggs, & Wise, 2012). This relationship existed even after controlling for lifestyle factors.

Research in perinatal health suggests that Black women may have more lifetime exposure to trauma, and this directly affects their rates of preterm birth. For example, in a national survey of 1,581 pregnant women (709 were Black women), there was more lifetime PTSD and trauma exposure for Black women (Seng, Kohn-Wood, McPherson, & Sperlich, 2011). Current prevalence for PTSD was 4 times higher for Black women. The rates did not differ by SES and are explained by greater trauma exposure. Child abuse was the most common cause of PTSD for both groups.

High rates of trauma and PTSD during pregnancy are concerning because of their relationship to both low birthweight and gestational age. A prospective, 3-cohort sample of first-time pregnant women compared 255 women with PTSD; 307 trauma-exposed, resilient women (no PTSD); and 277 non-trauma-exposed women (Seng, Low, Sperlich, Ronis, & Liberzon, 2011). They found that babies born to PTSD+ women weighed 283 g less than those born to resilient women and 221 g less than those born to non-exposed women. PTSD was also associated with a shorter gestation. These findings suggest trauma exposure and PTSD in pregnancy increased the risk for preterm birth, and both are more common in Black women.

Inflammation is a possible mechanism for this relationship. A study of mothers with stress and depression revealed high levels of the inflammatory molecules IL-6 and TNF-alpha (Coussons-Read, 2005). In addition to fighting infections and healing wounds, these molecules also ripen the cervix, increasing the likelihood of preterm birth. Along these same lines, a randomized clinical trial using DHA-enhanced eggs also suggest that inflammation is related to preterm birth (Smuts, 2003).

In this trial, 291 mothers were asked to eat one egg a day for the last trimester of their pregnancies. The eggs were either regular or were enriched with the omega-3 fatty acid DHA. DHA is highly anti-inflammatory. The mothers were participating in the WIC program in Kansas City. Approximately 70% of the sample was African American. This simple, cheap intervention increased gestation length by 6 days.

How Shall We Then Treat?

Understanding the mechanism underlying health disparities gives us some possible places to intervene. While we continue to work for social justice in the wider society, there are ways we can intervene when working with a particular client or patient.

We must start by acknowledging the health effects of discrimination and recognizing how it contributes to health disparities. In fact, given these health effects, we might even argue that microaggressions rise to the status of trauma exposure (i.e., the body is perceiving that it these events are a physical threat).

To address preterm birth, we need to be proactive in screening for depression and PTSD in pregnancy. We also need to counter the effects of chronic inflammation directly by supplementing with omega-3 fatty acids (particularly DHA and EPA) (Kendall-Tackett, 2010a).

Most American women are deficient in these and they are safe to use in pregnant women (see Kendall-Tackett, 2009a). In postpartum women, breastfeeding downregulates the stress response and decreases inflammation. It is important to continue to support community organizations that are increasing breastfeeding rates in the African American community. This will help with the health of both mothers and babies (Groer & Kendall-Tackett, 2011).

Finally, we need to recommend activities that we know downregulate the stress and inflammatory response systems, including both exercise and long-chain omega-3s (Kendall-Tackett, 2009b). Both help and will improve the health of African Americans and hopefully decrease health disparities.

References

Beatty, D. L., Hall, M. H., Kamarck, T. W., Buysse, D. J., Owens, J. F., Reis, S. E., ... Matthews, K. A. (2011). Unfair treatment is associated with poor sleep in African American and Caucasian adults: Pittsburgh Sleep-SCORE Project. *Health Psychology, 30*(3), 351-359.

Boynton-Jarrett, R., Rosenberg, L., Palmer, J. R., Boggs, D. A., & Wise, L. A. (2012). Child and adolescent abuse in relation to obesity in adulthood: The Black Women's Health Study. *Pediatrics, 130*(2), 245-253.

Cappuccio, F. P., Taggart, F. M., Kandala, N. B., Currie, A., Peile, E., Stranges, S., & Miller, M. A. (2008). Meta-analysis of short sleep duration and obesity in children and adults. *Sleep, 31*(5), 19-26.

Centers for Disease Control and Prevention. (2014a). *Life expectancy at birth, by sex and race/ethnicity—United States,2011*. Retrieved from http://www.cdc.gov/nchs/data/nvsr/nvsr63/nvsr63_03.pdf

Centers for Disease Control and Prevention. (2014b). *Racial and ethnic differences in diagnosed diabetes among people aged 20 years or older, United States, 2010-2012*. Retrieved from http://www.cdc.gov/diabetes/pdfs/data/2014-report-national-diabetes-statistics-report-data-sources.pdf

Coussons-Read, M. E., Okun, M.L., Schmitt, M.P., & Giese, S. (2005). Prenatal stress alters cytokine levels in a manner that may endanger human pregnancy. *Psychosomatic Medicine, 67*, 625-631.

Danese, A., Moffitt, T. E., Harrington, H., Milne, B. J., Polanczyk, G., Pariante, C. M., & Caspi, A. (2009). Adverse childhood experiences and adult risk factors for age-related disease: Depression, inflammation, and clustering of metabolic risk factors. *Archives of Pediatric and Adolescent Medicine, 163*(12), 1135-1143.

Dickerson, S. S. (2011). Physiological responses to experiences of social pain. In G. MacDonald & L. A. Jensen-Campbell (Eds.), *Social pain: Neuropsychological and health implications of social loss and exclusion* (pp. 79-94). Washington, DC: American Psychological Association

Eisenberger, N. I. (2011). The neural basis of social pain: Findings and implications. In G. MacDonald & L. A. Jensen-Campbell (Eds.), *Social pain: Neuropsychological and health implications of loss and exclusions* (pp. 53-78). Washington, DC: American Psychological Association.

Goodman, E., McEwen, B. S., Huang, B., Dolan, L. M., & Adler, N. E. (2005). Social inequalities in biomarkers of cardiovascular risk in adolescence. *Psychosomatic Medicine, 67*, 9-15.

Groer, M. W., & Kendall-Tackett, K. A. (2011). *How breastfeeding protects women's health throughout the lifespan: The psychoneuroimmunology of human lactation*. Amarillo, TX: Hale Publishing.

Haffner, S., & Taegtmeyer, H. (2003). Epidemic obesity and the metabolic syndrome. *Circulation, 108*, 1541-1545.

Hall, M. H., Muldoon, M. F., Jennings, J. R., Buysse, D. J., Flory, J. D., & Manuck, S. B. (2008). Self-reported sleep duration is associated with the metabolic syndrome in midlife adults. *Sleep, 31*(5), 635-643.

Hong, S., Nelesen, R. A., Krohn, P. L., Mills, P. J., & Dimsdale, J. E. (2006). The association of social status and blood pressure with markers of vascular inflammation. *Psychosomatic Medicine, 68*, 517-523.

Jenson-Campbell, L. A., & MacDonald, G. (2011). Introduction: Experiencing the ache of social injuries--an integrative approach to understanding social pain. In G. MacDonald & L. A. Jensen-Campbell (Eds.), *Social pain: Neuropsychological and health implications of loss and exclusino* (pp. 3-8). Washington, DC: American Psychological Association.

Kendall-Tackett, K. A. (2009a). Can fats make you happy? Depression and long-chain Omega-3 fatty acids in the perinatal period. *Medications and More, 38*(1), 1-2.

Kendall-Tackett, K. A. (2009b). Psychological trauma and physical health: A psychoneuroimmunology approach to etiology of negative heatlh effects and possible interventions. *Psychological Trauma, 1*(1), 35-48.

Kendall-Tackett, K. A. (2010a). Long-chain omega-3 fatty acids and women's mental health in the perinatal period. *Journal of Midwifery and Women's Health, 55*(6), 561-567.

Kendall-Tackett, K. A. (Ed.). (2010b). *The psychoneuroimmunology of chronic disease.* Washington, DC: American Psychological Association.

Lewis, T. T., Everson-Rose, S. A., Powell, L. H., Matthews, K. A., Brown, C., Karavolos, K., et al. (2006). Chronic exposure to everyday discrimination and coronary artery calcification in African American women: The SWAN Heart Study. *Psychosomatic Medicine, 68,* 362-368.

McDade, T. W., Hawkley, L. C., & Cacioppo, J. T. (2006). Psychosocial and behavioral predictors of inflammation in middle-aged and older adults: The Chicago Health, Aging, and Social Relations Study. *Psychosomatic Medicine, 68,* 376-381.

McEwen, B. S. (2003). Mood disorders and allostatic load. *Biological Psychiatry, 54,* 200-207.

Mezick, E. J., Matthews, K. A., Hall, M., Strollo, P. J., Buysse, D. J., Kamarck, T. W., ... Reis, S. E. (2008). Influence of race and socioeconomic status on sleep: Pittsburgh Sleep-SCORE Project. *Psychosomatic Medicine, 70,* 410-416.

Panksepp, J. (2011). The neurobiology of social loss in animals: Some keys to the puzzle of psychic pain in humans. In G. MacDonald & L. A. Jensen-Campbell (Eds.), *Social pain: Neuropsychological and health implications of loss and exclusion* (pp. 11-51). Washington, DC: American Psychological Association.

Rich-Edwards, J. W., Spiegelman, D., Hibert, E. N. L., Jun, H.-J., Todd, T. J., Kawachi, I., & Wright, R. J. (2010). Abuse in childhood and adolescence as a predictor of type-2 diabetes in adult women. *American Journal of Preventive Medicine, 39*(6), 529-536.

Seng, J. S., Kohn-Wood, L. P., McPherson, M. D., & Sperlich, M. A. (2011). Disparity in posttraumatic stress disorder diagnosis among African American pregnant women. *Archives of Women's Mental Health, 14*(4), 295-306.

Seng, J. S., Low, L. K., Sperlich, M. A., Ronis, D. L., & Liberzon, I. (2011). Posttraumatic stress disorder, child abuse history, birth weight, and gestational age: A prospective cohort study. *British Journal of Obstetrics & Gynecology, 118*(11), 1329-1339.

Slopen, N., Lewis, T. T., Gruenewald, T. L., Mujahid, M. S., Ryff, C. D., Albert, M. A., & Williams, D. R. (2010). Early life adversity and inflammation in African Americans and whites in midlife in the United States Survey. *Psychosomatic Medicine, 72,* 694-701.

Smuts, C. M., Huang, M., Mundy, D., Plasse, T., Major, S., & Carlson, S.E. (2003). A randomized trial of docosahexaenoic acid supplementation during the third trimester of pregnancy. *Obstetrics & Gynecology, 101,* 469-479.

Suarez, E. C., & Goforth, H. (2010). Sleep and inflammation: A potential link to chronic diseases. In K. A. Kendall-Tackett (Ed.), *The psychoneuroimmunology of chronic disease* (pp. 53-75). Washington, DC: American Psychological Association.

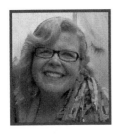

Kathleen Kendall-Tackett, PhD, IBCLC, RLC, FAPA, is past-President of the APA Division of Trauma Psychology and a Fellow in both trauma and health psychology. She is the Owner and Editor-in-Chief of Praeclarus Press, a small press specializing in women's health, and Editor-in-Chief of the journals *Clinical Lactation* and *Psychological Trauma.* This article was the Presidential Address to the Division of Trauma Psychology of the American Psychological Association in 2014.

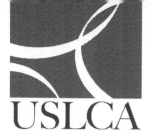

Free to Breastfeed: Voices of Black Mothers

A Book, a Website, a Movement

Barbara D. Robertson, MA, IBCLC, RLC[1]

Keywords: Black mothers, African American mothers, breastfeeding, racism

Anayah R. Sangodele-Ayoka and Jeanine Valrie Logan are the creators of Brown Mamas Breastfeed, an online campaign to promote the visibility of African American women who breastfeed, and have just released their book, Free to Breastfeed: Voices from Black Mothers, based on that work. Barbara D. Robertson interviews Anayah and Jeanine about their work and their experiences as breastfeeding mothers and what they hope to accomplish with their Free-to-Breastfeed project. They also describe some of the barriers to breastfeeding that Black

---

1   barbara@bfcaa.com

women encounter, and what lactation consultants can do to support Black women in their communities and in their profession.

Barbara: How did the two of you meet?

Jeanine: Anayah and I met online. We are both from Chicago and have a couple of mutual friends. We were introduced on Facebook because of our common interest and goal of becoming midwives. We both had our first child in 2010 and began to communicate about common parenting practices. It's really funny because the first time we met in person was in summer 2011, after we had already did the *Brown Mamas Breastfeed* online project. Technology is amazing.

Barbara: Why did you feel the calling to create *Free to Breastfeed: Voices of Black Mothers*?

Jeanine: The idea to create *Free to Breastfeed: Voices of Black Mothers* was actually the result and afterthought of the *Brown Mamas Breastfeed* project. We are both bloggers. Anayah reached out to me about a post I wrote and suggested that we do an online project with both of our blogs highlighting Black breastfeeding mamas and why they love breastfeeding. This was launched on Mother's Day 2011. It was a project to inundate the Internet with beautiful photos of Black breastfeeding moms. We put a call out to our online communities and, needless to say, we got a great response, with over 5,000 hits on our individual websites.

Anayah: We had become parents for the first time, and breastfeeding added a whole other layer... realizing the gravity and opportunity that breastfeeding can be with the bonding and personal empowerment, as well as the health benefits, of course, for mother and baby. We were both dismayed that we didn't see much diversity in the images of women breastfeeding. We would get calls from people looking for diverse images ... and we could say, "Hey, here are some!" We made them available for people. We just ask them for us to credit us.

Almost every one of the women also included a more lengthy narrative. We were struck by what was an obvious desire to be heard as well as seen. It got us thinking about how the attention to disparities in breastfeeding rates can be disempowering to African American women. *Free to Breastfeed* makes the case for considering for viewing Black women as complex human beings and individuals rather than a population with a problem needing to be fixed by others.

As we continued the project, we found ourselves becoming breastfeeding advocates on a larger scale than just in our personal circle. We found we could have a greater impact by continuing to produce materials tha told the Black breast-feeding woman's story. The book has been basically born from that (Figure 1). We are planning on having a really big launch that will include a lot of virtual events. It will be fun and informative and just have opportunities for people to connect.

Figure 1. *Free to Breastfeed* book cover.

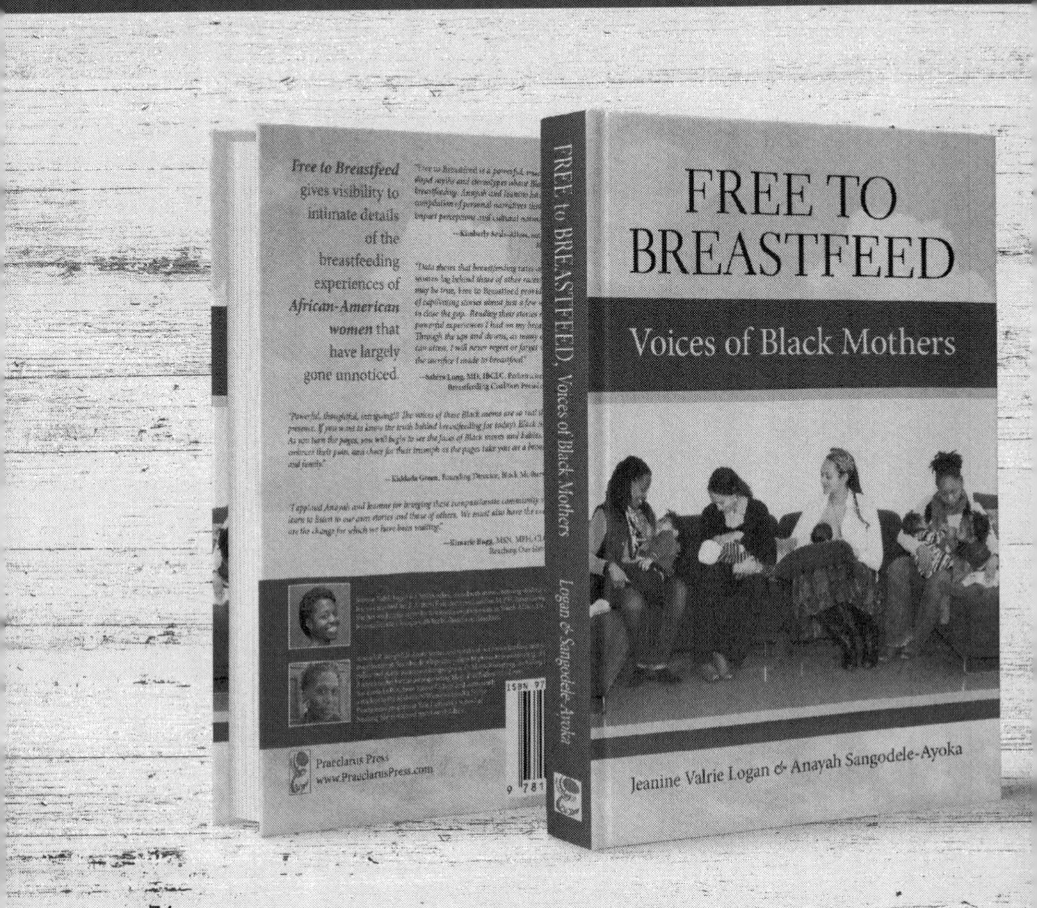

Barbara: Where is the best place to find out about these events? Your website?

Jeanine: Our website, our Facebook page, our Twitter page. We have been working so hard on the book so not much else has been happening. We are keeping the website updated with everything. People can join our email list through the website for more information. We will be in local venues, too, so people can come out in person, meet the authors, get a book signed, and meet mamas—breastfeeding mamas.

Barbara: So, you didn't start out to write a book. You started out wanting to diversify the images, but then it turned into a book.

Anayah: When people sent us their images, we asked people to answer three questions:

1. How long have you breastfeed?

2. Why did you breastfeed?

3. Why is it important for you, as a Black mother, to breastfeed?

They were simple questions, but we found that the responses were really poignant and eloquent. So we expanded the project for a call for narratives, poetry, stories, and photos. The response was greater than I thought we were going to get back.

Jeanine: The images and the videos that we put on YouTube went viral. Just from those couple of things that we did, so many people wanted to connect with us, and have us present at a workshop or anything like that. It really touched people. The more I looked at it, I realized there really wasn't anything like it on the market, as far as books that have an emphasis on Black women and breastfeeding. We have some that are technical, which is great, but they are more about how to breastfeed, and we think that is great, but feel that that information isn't really going to change much.

Barbara: What surprised you the most when gathering Black mother's breastfeeding stories?

Anayah: I've been most surprised by the latent breastfeeding advocate that seems to be hiding out in so many breastfeeding mothers. It's not difficult to find women who breastfed and want to spread the word to both celebrate their accomplishment and encourage other mothers. I think that's really phenomenal. These women are saying, "We *do* breastfeed!" and see *Free to Breastfeed* as an opportunity to help support other moms they may never meet to do the same. Also, a lot of the women were really compassionate and vocal about not shaming women who didn't or couldn't breastfeed. That awareness was also really touching to me.

Barbara: Why stories, not statistics?

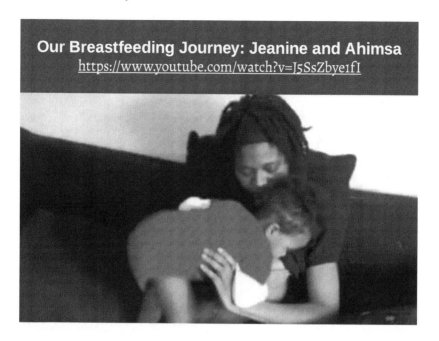

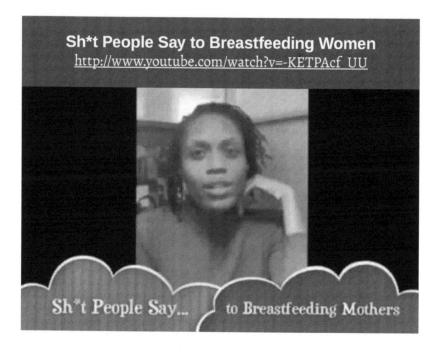

Jeanine: Stories—that's a different level of connection and impact. The narrative is that Black women don't breastfeed, but rarely is the narrative actually from Black women. Rarely do we hear our stories of why we did or why we didn't try. So we just really wanted to create a space where we could talk about breastfeeding from a place of empowerment, and not from a space where we are waiting for something else to happen or waiting for somebody else to initiate it. It's really surprising that, even in the 3 years that we have been doing this, more visibility is being made. Sisters are making the way for Black women and breastfeeding to be on the front lines, lots of initiatives, and programming. This is the only book, or the only place, you will find that is talking about our culture and talking about our legacy, history, and families—things that are empowering our communities. However, these women came to breastfeed—or love breastfeeding—they are doing something revolutionary as both as mothers and community members.

You can read about statistics anywhere, and more specifically, stats about how Black women in America are the least likely to initiate breastfeeding, and for those that do, the duration is shorter. What you don't see or hear is any acknowledgment on the shift in the current trend with more Black women initiating breastfeeding. You don't hear about these mamas that are creating a cultural shift. You don't hear about the activism and advocacy that Black women are doing to change the highly visible, predominantly White breastfeeding culture. You won't easily read about our breastfeeding legacies and cultural wisdom as it pertains to breastfeeding. The world never hears our narratives and our stories since many of them are being written for us. All of these things are why I see this book as more of a book about agency, resilience, commitment, and empowerment. However, whatever moved these women to come to breastfeeding, these are acts of revolution and resilience that will radically change their families and their communities in the most fundamental way.

Barbara: On your website, you each use the word *justice*. Anayah, your bio says *reproductive justice*, and Jeanine, you use the words *birth justice*. What do you mean by those words?

Jeanine: Birth justice is a newer term that has evolved from the tenets of the *reproductive justice* movement. [A Black women's caucus first coined the term reproductive justice, naming themselves Women of African Descent for Reproductive Justice at the Illinois Pro-Choice Alliance Conference in Cairo, Egypt in November 1994 to begin to address the specific needs of Black women.] Birth justice is part of this larger movement and acts to resist reproductive oppressions. It looks at the intersections of gender, race, class, sexuality, etc. and how our places in these social domains are directly and intentionally related to our poor experiences surrounding birth. Birth justice continues to address racism within the medical industrial complex, the prison industrial complex, and other institutional systems that influence and fuel inequities in the birth outcomes of women of color, especially for Black women. Lastly, birth justice also works to increase access to culturally specific birth care; breastfeeding support; and the right to choose if, when, and how many babies we want. When I speak of birth justice, I speak of reproductive justice as well.

Barbara: Were you two breastfed yourselves? How did you become breastfeeding women?

Anayah: I was. I come from a breastfeeding family.

Jeanine: I was actually not breastfed myself. I tell my story in the *Foreword* of the book. It is actually my mother's story. She had very dense breast tissue, and very cystic breasts, and began having surgeries to remove the cysts when she was 12 or 13 years old. So by the time she had me 10 years later, at that time, it was in the '70s and physicians were saying she should not breastfeed because it might actually increase her risk for breast cancer. Now, obviously, that's not true. So she didn't breastfeed me, and hearing her tell that story throughout my childhood, she was always saying that *this information that I got was wrong. So when you have your children, you really should think about doing this.* My mom died when she was 43 years old from breast cancer. Now I am 36 and I can't imagine being dead in a few years, and not having the opportunity to do something as simple as nurse my children, or have someone discourage me to doing that, and at the end of the day still get cancer. That's been one of my biggest commitments—encouraging Black women to do this.

Barbara: We know that breast cancer rates are very high in Black women, and yet we don't really hear the breast cancer people talking about prevention. They talk about cures.

Jeanine: Oh my gosh, this really gets under my skin because we know that even up until recently, we were talking about Black women dying of the most aggressive forms of breast cancer because we weren't getting screened as regularly, but we know now that that's not even the case. Even screening is not as preventative as it was thought to be. But it really bothers me that, I think the breast cancer, I don't want to call it the breast cancer industry, that whole market around *curing* breast cancer, which is really great. We need a cure for breast cancer, but I think there's a really powerful opportunity there, especially in the African American community to talk about one of the few things that is within our control to prevent breast cancer that we know of, which is breastfeeding. We are missing a powerful opportunity that could really help us. When breastfeeding is discussed in the media, we are really allowing the conversation to be dominated by discussions of breastfeeding being a lifestyle choice when, for us, our work is really centered on saving Black women's lives, saving babies' lives. There is such an opportunity there, especially with breast cancer, to take stand or having a powerful voice to move breastfeeding forward in African American communities that's not being taken, and I wish it was. It all motivates our work!

Barbara: A lot of people who are not Black have a lot of ideas about how to help Black mothers be more successful with breastfeeding. Where are they going wrong?

Jeanine: Anytime a person sets their intentions on helping someone without inviting that someone to speak about their own perception of their needs, it becomes a recipe for disaster. I believe the best intentions don't make up for non-inclusivity and the continued disregard of the voices of women of color in the breastfeeding world. Not only does this happen with breastfeeding, but also within the entire birth culture world. Some organizations are getting hip and reaching out to Black people to understand their role in advocating for Black women. But there is still a long way to go. Realistically, there needs to be more women of color— and especially Black IBCLCs and birth workers—trained to support Black women in meeting their breastfeeding goals. This may mean that allies offer to mentor Black women and support their trainings by offering more scholarships, etc. Whatever the help is, it cannot exclude the Black mother's voice, what she feels she needs to better herself as a mother and community member.

Barbara: How can IBCLCs best support Black women?

Anayah: Again, I don't only think that this work is done in isolation. There are many gatekeepers along the road to breastfeeding success. Since oftentimes, it does start with the IBCLC, to start off, there has to be more IBCLCs of color. Until that happens, there has to be an increase in the number of ones that work within Black communities, ones that will make home visits, ones that offer sliding scale or free services. The peer counselor is an amazing role, usually someone that lives within community. We also have to utilize these women as they are supporting mothers on the margins; modeling breastfeeding success; as well as offering tangible, profession skills within their communities.

Jeanine: An IBCLC can mentor. They can help provide shadowing so that women of color can get those 1,000 [clinical] hours, provide educational opportunities or trainings for peer counselors. Not everyone needs to be an IBCLC, but there needs to be more people in communities who know how to support breastfeeding. Doing small things can be really important.

Anayah: Providing continuity of care, having care be seamless ... having more internships in community settings ... being involved in the community, community groups, Baby Cafes ... taking opportunities to develop cultural competencies. I know this term is being thrown around a lot but there are some excellent programs.

Kiddada Green, with the Black Mother's Breast-feeding Association, has great trainings. In a clinical setting, you have to be able to really think about that woman's life, her economic situation, her family situation and be able to think through those things and how do they relate to you as a clinical provider. You need to be able to understand someone on a human level, not just as a demographic, not the statistics.

Anayah: Most women are going to face social and cultural barriers. They may be in her own family. They may be doubting her supply. Not seeing other mothers breastfeeding, bad information, someone saying she needs to toughen up her nipples with a brush.

Jeanine: I do think that the health profession is very heavy in White population. When I took my breastfeeding training, we had about 500 people in the room; there were three IBCLCs. They had wonderful PowerPoints and were very professional. But for the whole 5 days, when anything came up about culture, they would say, very irresponsibly, with no second thought, *Well, you know, Black women don't particularly breastfeed, so you might have a struggle with that.*

And there I was, my baby was 4 months old, in the third row, pumping all day long for my Black baby, with my Black-woman self. And I was like, wow! That was the first time I had heard Black women don't breastfeed because here I was, doing it. I guess I don't count. I felt like those statements were racist; those statements were culturally insensitive. And they were irresponsible to tell a room of 500 lactation professionals that as you grow in your career, don't worry so much about the Black woman because they aren't going to breastfeed anyway. They were uncultured around the perceived needs for what women that look like me need. Professions that don't have a lot of diversity in them provide a framework that you are going to operate from which, in turn, can be experienced as very racist, very biased. When you have people who are working from these gazes that have nothing to do with the people they are serving, even the best intentions are void. You can go in there with a mentality of doing some good work, but if you are still operating from this predisposed ideology that is breed in America, then you are going to be very culturally insensitive, and in turn, do and say some pretty racist things.

Barbara: So perhaps the profession is perpetuating the myth, and making it stronger, that Black women don't breastfeed?

Anayah: We know that when our healthcare providers have low expectations, those expectations matter. Low expectations are real ... As a student nurse, my role as a professional is one of educating. A nurse is supposed to educate and empower her patients to see themselves as in control of their health and making the best decisions possible. And so we can't simultaneously hold that as a thought while saying it's not going to work anyway, so you just do what you can. We do have to be concerned with racial equity. Make sure mothers have the confidence and the support they need to be successful at breastfeeding; that has to be our mission. [We need to] remove whatever barriers; if those barriers exist as yourself, then you have to address that.

When we go to the ILCA 2014 Conference, at the Breastfeeding Summit, one of the topics that will be addressed is if you know that your profession isn't diverse enough—and research shows that this is important for the health of those communities that you want to serve—we need to do something about that. Then it is important for your organization to do something.

On a basic level, and it's not easy for anyone. You have to become comfortable with the dynamics of power shifting, with being uncomfortable at times, with being challenged about what you believe, or things that you have never actually thought about. It's going to be very uncomfortable, but I think it can be done. But I think that whether your organization is racist is the last question that should probably be asked because it shuts the door. Yes, we are racist. Or no, we are not racist. There's no place to go from there. The key is to think critically about how we can move forward and serve the population as it deserves to be served.

Jeanine: Saying someone is racist is such a reactionary way to look at the problem. Being proactive is to really be intentional. We need concrete goals. For example, by this year, we will have X number more women of color certified as IBCLCs.

Anayah: I am on the board of LEARC. We need to go to the community colleges and approach them about how we can do this [help low-income women with the college courses required to become an IBCLC]. We need to go to the communities where these women are and help make pathways for them. We have to go outside of what we have always done.

Barbara: What is your vision for Black mothers and breastfeeding in the United States?

Jeanine: I envision more social support for Black women to be able to start and continue their breast-feeding journeys. Research has shown that by the time a woman is 12 weeks pregnant, she has already made the decision whether or not she will breastfeed. I envision all providers using these opportunities to speak to Black women about the how to create that social support at home and within her community.

I envision more Black IBCLCs and peer counselors. I envision more women finding and accessing the support they need to reach their breastfeeding goals. Lastly, I hope that *Free to Breastfeed* finds its way into the hands of a woman that hadn't thought about breastfeeding and that it encourages her to do so. I envision more visibility for Black women. It's really that simple.

Anayah: My vision is that every Black woman has witnessed positive breastfeeding experiences prior to becoming a mother, has competent and compassionate support people she knows she can count on, and economic stability and paid family leave to spend time transitioning into parenthood with a real opportunity to grow into the new parent–child relationship through breastfeeding.

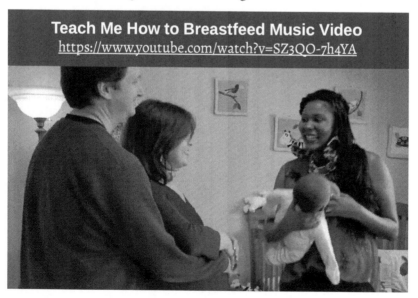

Teach Me How to Breastfeed Music Video
https://www.youtube.com/watch?v=SZ3QO-7h4YA

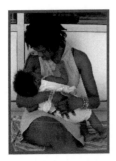

Jeanine Valrie Logan is a birthworker, homebirth mama, nursing student, and future midwife. Jeanine received her BA from Fisk University and an MPH from George Washington University. She has worked for reproductive justice organizations in South Africa, DC, and Chicago. Jeanine lives in Chicago with her husband and daughter.

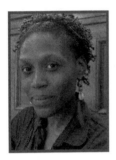

Anayah R. Sangodele-Ayoka writes and speaks about breastfeeding, maternal health, and personal empowerment. She also develops campaigns to promote breastfeeding-friendly communities through policy and public awareness campaigns with MomsRising. org, including Black Breastfeeding Week. Anayah writes for the corresponding blog www.freetobreastfeed.com). She earned a BA from Vassar College, and is currently a student in the Midwifery/Women's Health Nurse Practitioner program at Yale University School of Nursing. She is married with two children.

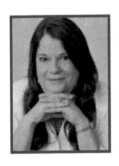

Barbara D. Robertson, MA, IBCLC, RLC, is the owner of The Breastfeeding Center of Ann Arbor, and an associate editor of *Clinical Lactation*. Barbara was director of professional development for the U.S. Lactation Consultant Association from 2009 to 2014. She received the Michigan Breastfeeding Network Outstanding Community Breastfeeding Support Award in 2009.

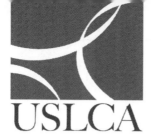

Social Support Improves Breastfeeding Self-Efficacy in a Sample of Black Women

Deborah McCarter-Spaulding, PhD, RN, IBCLC, RLC[1]
Rebecca Gore, PhD[2]

Keywords: Black women, self-efficacy, social support, network support

Black women in the United States have lower rates of initiation and duration of breastfeeding compared to other racial/ethnic groups. Social support for breastfeeding, as well as breastfeeding self-efficacy, has been reported as an influence on breastfeeding outcomes. This study analyzes the relationship between breastfeeding self-efficacy and network support for breastfeeding in a sample of Black women. Results showed that network

1   dmccarter@anselm.edu, Saint Anselm College, Manchester, NH
2   Rebecca_Gore@uml.edu, University of Massachusetts, Lowell

support for breastfeeding does not have a direct effect on breastfeeding duration and pattern, but it does have a significant influence on breastfeeding self-efficacy. These results provide theoretical support for clinical interventions designed to enhance the support network as a way of improving breastfeeding self-efficacy, particularly for women at risk for early weaning.

The good news is that breastfeeding rates are on the rise in the United States (McDowell et al., 2008). However, there are still significant demographic and racial differences in breastfeeding rates. Black women in the United States are less likely to initiate and continue breastfeeding (Ahluwalia et al., 2005). It is well accepted that many different psychosocial factors influence breastfeeding initiation, duration, and pattern. Understanding these influences can help to direct interventions to promote breastfeeding, particularly in groups at risk for never initiating breastfeeding, or for early weaning.

Breastfeeding self-efficacy is defined as a mother's belief that she will be able to organize and carry out the actions necessary to breastfeed her infant. Higher levels of breastfeeding self-efficacy have been shown to predict longer and more exclusive breastfeeding in varied samples of women (Blyth et al., 2002; Dai & Dennis, 2003; Gregory et al., 2008; Wutke & Dennis, 2007), including in a sample of Black women in the United States (McCarter-Spaulding & Gore, 2009). In addition, social support for breastfeeding is known to influence breastfeeding in either a positive or negative direction (McInnes & Chambers, 2008; Raj & Plichta, 1998).

Breastfeeding self-efficacy and social support have a theoretical relationship based on Bandura's Social Cognitive Theory (Bandura, 1997). Using this theory as a framework, a person's perception of self-efficacy is influenced by information received from various sources. One such source is vicarious experience, which can be understood as having appropriate role models. Another source of efficacy information is social or verbal persuasion, which can be understood as emotional support and encouragement. A social support network for breastfeeding can provide these sources of efficacy information and theoretically influence a woman's perception of her ability to successfully breastfeed her infant. In this study, breastfeeding-specific social support is measured by the Network Support for Breastfeeding (NSB) instrument, in which network support for breastfeeding is defined as the existence and quantity of social network available for a breastfeeding mother, and the functional quality of those relationships related specifically to breastfeeding support.

Perception of Self-Efficacy Is Influenced by Information from Various Sources, Including

- Vicarious experience, such as role models

- Social or verbal persuasion, such as emotional support and encouragement

---

In light of the significant racial disparities in breast-feeding rates, and the importance of breastfeeding to health, particularly for Black infants (Forste et al., 2001), a study was conducted measuring both breastfeeding self-efficacy and the network support for breastfeeding in a sample of Black women. The results of the analysis of breastfeeding self-efficacy to breastfeeding outcomes is reported elsewhere (McCarter-Spaulding & Gore, 2009). The current study is a report of the analysis of the network support for breastfeeding in the same sample. The purpose of the study was to determine if higher levels of social support predicted longer duration or more exclusive breastfeeding, particularly when breastfeeding self-efficacy was also taken into account.

Methods

Study Participants and Recruitment

The research was conducted in a large teaching hospital in the Northeast United States, with approval from the hospital's Institutional Review Board. The target population was breastfeeding Black women, defined as women who identified themselves as being of African descent, including the ethnic backgrounds of African, African American, Cape Verdean, Haitian, West Indian/ Caribbean, and Black Hispanic.

A convenience sample of Black women (N=155) was recruited during their postpartum hospitalization from three maternity units of a large urban teaching hospital.

Breastfeeding was defined as any feedings at the breast in the past 24 hours, or if the baby had not been fed, the reported intention to breastfeeding.

Participants were healthy women aged 18 or older who were able to read and speak English, and had given birth to healthy singleton infants at 37 weeks gestation or greater.

The mean age of the women participating in the study was 30.4 (SD = 6.5, range 18 to 45). The majority of participants (68.3%) was either married or living with a partner. Most of the respondents (96.7%) had a minimum of a high school education. The majority had delivered vaginally (66%) and was multiparous (58%). Of those who reported their incomes, the largest proportion of the sample (32%) reported a household income of $81,000/year or higher, but more than half of the sample (54%) reported a household income of less than $40,000/year. In addition, 58% of the sample reported eligibility for participation in the Women, Infants and Children program (WIC), which considers both household income and number of household members.

A majority of the respondents had worked outside the home in the year prior to their pregnancy (83%), and their incomes generally represented up to one half of the household income.

Instruments

During the hospitalization, and again at one month postpartum, respondents completed the Breastfeeding

Self-Efficacy Scale, Short Form (BSES-SF) (Dennis, 2003), as well as the investigator-developed Network Support for Breastfeeding (NSB) instrument.

The Network Support for Breastfeeding (NSB) instrument was designed based on review of the literature, clinical experience and consultation with colleagues. It measures the existence and quantity of the network support available in the context of breastfeeding, and the functional quality of those relationships related to breastfeeding support for five to seven individuals in the social network, as well as the professionals in the hospital and primary care setting. The instrument was pretested, content validity was established, and analysis using Cronbach's alpha showed a reliability coefficient of 0.87-.90. Scores were calculated based on average support from each person in the network, and could range from 0 to 3.

At each month postpartum, respondents were also asked about their breastfeeding pattern. Mothers reported the number and method of feedings in the previous 24 hours, and their responses were categorized according to Labbok and Krasovec's (1990) six categories of breastfeeding. Feeding expressed mother's milk in a bottle was coded as *breastfeeding*. The responses were then combined into three categories for statistical analysis: breastfeeding exclusively, combination of breastfeeding and formula-feeding, or formula-feeding only. They were also asked whether they had returned to work or school during that month. Participants were followed monthly until 6 months postpartum or until complete weaning [cessation of breastfeeding].

Results

Characteristics of Network Support

Based on the NSB scoring system, most participants had a higher-than-average perception of breastfeeding support. Support from the women's mother was rated the highest, followed by partners and friends.

The average number of support people for each respondent was 5 (SD = 1). Women with previous breastfeeding experience reported a slightly lower perception of support (support score = 2.2) compared to those who were breastfeeding for the first time (support score = 2.3), but this difference was not statistically significant. The average support from the pediatric providers was 2.8 (SD = 0.45, range 0 to 3).

Relationship of Network Support to Breastfeeding Outcomes

Higher level of network support for breastfeeding as measured by the NSB did not predict breastfeeding pattern or duration either independently or when breastfeeding self-efficacy was included as a variable in the regression analysis. However, when network support for breastfeeding was entered into a linear regression analysis with breastfeeding self-efficacy as the outcome, it significantly predicted breastfeeding self-efficacy, such that higher levels of support were predictive of higher levels of breastfeeding self-efficacy.

Discussion

While network support for breastfeeding did not predict breastfeeding outcomes when breastfeeding self-efficacy was taken into consideration, the level of network support for breastfeeding predicted the level of breastfeeding self-efficacy, consistent with self-efficacy theory (Bandura, 1997). As network support for breastfeeding is potentially modifiable, this provides good theoretical support for interventions that enhance a woman's support network in ways that will improve her breastfeeding self-efficacy, beginning with an assessment of the level of breastfeeding support that she is expecting to receive from her social network.

If breastfeeding is not the social norm, support for breastfeeding may need to be sought outside the existing social network. This may be the case for Black mothers, as they may be making the decision to breastfeed in the absence of role models and family support (Ludington-Hoe et al., 2002).

Mothers can be referred to community resources, such as La Leche League groups, or breastfeeding support groups. However, based on self-efficacy theory (Bandura, 1997), mothers need to find role models that they judge as similar to themselves in order for such influences to improve their perception of their ability to be successful. This may mean that careful consideration should be made as to which support groups may or may not provide the desired effect.

Nurses and lactation consultants may want to guide mothers to supportive networks, such as peer counseling through WIC, or informal connections with experienced mothers who are similar to them and who could provide role modeling for the unfamiliar experience of breastfeeding. Creating support groups for women who see themselves as peers may be appropriate, rather than referring all women to the same sources of support.

Taking the time to do an intentional inventory of where to find support in one's social network can help women to identify new relationships that may need to be developed in order to be successful in their breastfeeding goals.

Conclusion

To those experienced with supporting breastfeeding mothers, it is not new news that supportive relationships can help women to achieve their breastfeeding goals. However, understanding the theoretical underpinnings of this mechanism helps us plan interventions knowing that research evidence supports what clinicians have known intuitively through experience. Knowing that network support appears to influence mothers through the mechanism of improving self-efficacy suggests that it is but one tool among many that can improve self-efficacy.

It is also important to confirm that breastfeeding self-efficacy and network support for breastfeeding influence breastfeeding in this sample of Black women, similar to other racial/ethnic groups. Using findings from diverse groups of women is important to establish culturally appropriate interventions based on evidence. Breastfeeding self-efficacy has been shown to be a robust predictor of breastfeeding duration and pattern, and developing interventions based on this theory will help us meet the nation's breastfeeding goals (American Academy of Pediatrics, 2005), and to plan research toward the same end. Working to improve the social network for breastfeeding support is one important and viable way to accomplish these goals.

References

Ahluwalia, I. B., Morrow, B., & Hsia, J. (2005). Why do women stop breastfeeding? Findings from the Pregnancy Risk Assessment and Monitoring System. *Pediatrics, 116*(6), 1408-1412.

American Academy of Pediatrics. (2005). Breastfeeding and the use of human milk. *Pediatrics, 115*(2), 496-506.

Bandura, A. (1997). *Self-efficacy: The exercise of control.* New York: W.H. Freeman and Company.

Blyth, R., Creedy, D. K., Dennis, C., Moyle, W., Pratt, J., & De Vries, S. M. (2002). Effect of maternal confidence on breastfeeding duration: An application of breastfeeding selfefficacy theory. *Birth: Issues in Perinatal Care, 29*(4), 278-274.

Dai, X., & Dennis, C. (2003). Translation and validation of the Breastfeeding Self-Efficacy Scale into Chinese. *Journal of Midwifery & Women's Health, 48*(5), 350-356.

Dennis, C. (2003). The Breastfeeding Self-Efficacy Scale: Psychometric assessment of the short form. *JOGNN, 32*(6), 734-744.

Forste, R., Weiss, J., & Lippincott, E. (2001). The decision to breastfeed in the United States: Does race matter? *Pediatrics, 108*(2), 291-296.

Gregory, A., Penrose, K., Morrison, C., Dennis, C., & MacArthur, C. (2008). Psychometric properties of the Breastfeeding Self-Efficacy Scale-Short Form in an ethnically diverse U.K. sample. *Public Health Nursing, 25*(3), 278-284.

Labbok, M., & Krasovec, K. (1990). Toward consistency in breastfeeding definitions. *Studies in Family Planning, 21*(4), 226-230.

Ludington-Hoe, S. M., McDonald, P. E., & Satyshur, R. (2002). Breastfeeding in African-American Women. *Journal of the National Black Nurses Association, 13*(1), 56-64.

McCarter-Spaulding, D., & Gore, R. (2009). Breastfeeding self-efficacy in women of African descent. *JOGNN, 38*(2), 230-243.

McDowell, M. A., Wang, C.-Y., & Kennedy-Stephenson, J. (2008). *Breastfeeding in the United States: Findings from the National Health and Nutrition Examination Surveys 1999-2006, NCHS data briefs, no 5.* Hyattsville, MD: National Center for Health Statistics.

McInnes, R. J., & Chambers, J. A. (2008). Supporting breastfeeding mothers: Qualitative synthesis. *Journal of Advanced Nursing, 62*(4), 407-427.

Raj, V. K., & Plichta, S. B. (1998). Literature review. The role of social support in breastfeeding promotion: A literature review. *Journal of Human Lactation, 14*(1), 41-45.

Wutke, K., & Dennis, C. (2007). The reliability and validity of the Polish version of the Breastfeeding Self-Efficacy Scale-Short Form: Translation and psychometric assessment. *International Journal of Nursing Studies, 44*(8), 1439-1446.

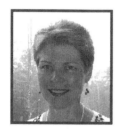
Deborah McCarter-Spaulding, PhD, WNHP-BC, RN, IBCLC, RLC, has been certified as a lactation consultant since 1989, and has cared for postpartum women and their infants for many years as a maternity nurse and as a Women's Health Nurse Practitioner. She is currently an Associate Professor at Saint Anselm College in Manchester, NH, where she teaches childbearing nursing in both the classroom and clinical settings. Her clinical experience has motivated her to research modifiable factors that can guide interventions to support women at risk for not breastfeeding or early weaning.

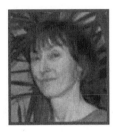 **Rebecca Gore, PhD,** is a Statistical Applications Programmer at the University of Massachusetts, Lowell, Department of Work Environment. Her experience as an employed breastfeeding mother, as well as her statistical expertise, helped guide her invaluable research support of Deborah McCarter-Spaulding's work with breastfeeding in Black women.

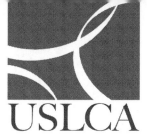

An Innovator in Lactation Equity

Q & A With Sherry Payne, MSN, RN, CNE, IBCLC, RLC

Marie Hemming, IBCLC, RLC[1]

Keywords: African American, health disparities, breastfeeding, infant mortality

Sherry Payne, MSN, RN, CNE, IBCLC, RLC, is the executive director of Uzazi Village, a nonprofit organization devoted to decreasing pregnancy-related health disparities in the urban core of Kansas City. She also facilitated the 2014 Lactation Summit: Addressing Inequities Within the Lactation Consultant Profession. *Ms. Payne speaks frequently around the country to professional audiences on topics related to lactation and birth disparities. One of the many barriers that aspiring International Board*

---

1   myhemming@gmail.com

Certified Lactation Consultants (IBCLCs) of color face is acquiring clinical hours. The Uzazi Village Lactation Consultant Mentorship Program is an innovative solution connecting aspiring IBCLCs from the Kansas City community to the Uzazi Village Breastfeeding Clinic, which provides free services to area families. Ms. Payne was recently interviewed by Marie Hemming, IBCLC, RLC, a member of the International Lactation Consultant Association's Medialert Team.

Marie Hemming: Why did you start the Lactation Consultant Mentorship Program?

Sherry Payne: I started this program with the idea that we needed more IBCLCs of color. I am currently the only IBCLC of color practicing in my city (though I am the third African American IBCLC to be certified in my community). This has become a top priority for Uzazi Village: making accessible pathways for lactation educators and peer counselors to become board-certified professionals, and then linking those professionals to families in our community who need those services. We already had our free breastfeeding clinic up and running 2 days a week, and four volunteer IBCLCs to run it. It was not too difficult to add the mentorship program to it. Three of our IBCLCs qualify to be mentors, and there were always plenty of women at our door inquiring about how to become lactation consultants. The research tells us that recruiting and diversifying the ranks of IBCLCs should be a part of the strategy for overcoming disparities in lactation in the African American community. That's what we are attempting to do.

Marie: **Tell us about the breastfeeding clinic and how it serves families in Kansas City.**

Sherry: Clients are referred from community-based prenatal clinics and local hospitals that serve low-income breastfeeding women who otherwise would not be able to the lactation support they need. I talk to the local lactation consultants, nurse midwives, pediatricians, doulas, and other care providers about our clinic. We receive referrals from Women, Infants, and Children (WIC) and home visiting programs, such as Healthy Start and Nurse Family Partnership. We have three to five moms in clinic, and home visits each day, and we spend an average of 2 hours with each client on everything from sore nipples, to milk supply issues, to relactation and weaning. We also offer two breastfeeding support groups: La Leche League on Troost and the Chocolate Milk Café. Our support groups and breastfeeding classes also draw local women into the clinic.

Marie: How does the mentorship program work?

Sherry: The interns need to accumulate 300 or 500 hours, and we ask that they work at the breastfeeding clinic a minimum of 1 day per week every other week. If they come to every clinic, it will take them 4–6 months, or it may take them as long as 10 months to get their hours if they come less often. They are also encouraged to take the WHO/UNICEF Breastfeeding course, which is offered every quarter. The interns pay a fee for the program on a sliding scale depending on income. The program is just starting out; however, we have our first intern beginning in May 2014, with two other candidates seeking placement. We are currently working on getting hospital placement for our interns to do part of their hours. We are also in talks with a local community college to package all the required courses to create a one-stop shopping curriculum for our interns. We hope to be able to simplify things by having classes and clinical experiences all in one program.

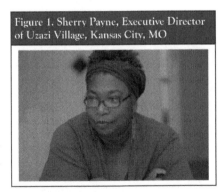

Figure 1. Sherry Payne, Executive Director of Uzazi Village, Kansas City, MO

Resource

Interview With Sherry Payne on Fighting Breastfeeding Disparities With Support, http://kcur.org/post/kc-group-fights-breast-feeding-disparities-education-support

Marie: What are some of the other barriers that aspiring IBCLCs of color experience? How is Uzazi Village helping to break down those barriers?

Sherry: Barriers for aspiring IBCLCs include accessing the educational components, finding mentors, and completing the hours. Women of color will of course be much less likely to find mentors that look like them, and normative culture mentors may be uncomfortable bringing a woman of color into their practice. (I am actually experiencing the same difficulty in my midwifery training.)

Many aspiring IBCLCs of color are found in the ranks of WIC peer counselors, but there is no clear cut pathway to move them into the ranks of IBCLCs. It is the presence of these types of barriers that compelled me to create a program at Uzazi Village. International Board of Lactation Consultant Examiners requirements often presuppose educational attainment that peer counselors may not possess, leaving them stranded at the bottom of the professional and economic rungs.

Marie: You were invited to Washington, DC, by the United States Breastfeeding Committee to discuss continuity of care with advocates from around the country. If you could change one thing about our healthcare system to improve breastfeeding outcomes, what would it be?

Sherry: The Affordable Care Act makes provision for reimbursement for lactation professionals. I would like to see reimbursement for *all* levels of breastfeeding support professionals: direct compensation for the work we do, particularly WIC peer counselors. We need our WIC peer counselors in our communities. Lactation consultants are most often isolated in hospitals, and accessing them is difficult, if not impossible, following hospital discharge. Private practice IBCLCs are cost prohibitive to access among the women we regularly see. Peer counselors have had the greatest impact on increasing breastfeeding rates in our community: They do most of the frontline work, and yet they receive the least amount of recognition and pay. I would like to see peer counselors and certified lactation counselors compensated by insurance companies for the valuable service and support they offer. This does not take anything away from the board-certified professional, but enhances and refines his or her role. We need all levels of expertise.

Marie: **Of all of the things that you have done, are there one or two things that stand out as being most effective in helping the moms that come to Uzazi Village?**

Sherry: The Chocolate Milk Café, which is a mother-to-mother support group for African American women, has been groundbreaking. It is designed to meet the needs of our urban moms and has been one of our most successful programs. At Chocolate Milk Café, mothers can attend with their babies and have a safe environment in which to discuss their breast-feeding issues. We are starting to replicate this model around the country.

Marie: **You are breaking new ground with your work at Uzazi Village; is there someone who has influenced you or mentored you in your own career as a lactation consultant and natural birth educator?**

Sherry: Lots of people have invested in my success over the years, but my primary mentor in lactation has been Charlene Burnett, BSN, RN, IBCLC, RLC. She mentored me when I was an L & D nurse, but I worked at a different hospital. She received special permission from her hospital to mentor me 500 hours in a year. I could not have done this without her. She is one of my LC volunteers, and she is the director of Lactation Services at Uzazi Village. We have named a scholarship after her: the Charlene L. M. Burnett IBCLC Scholarship, set aside for a candidate of color in the greater metropolitan area of Kansas, Missouri, who has met all requirements to sit for the IBLCE exam. It is our small way of thanking her for all that she has invested in Uzazi Village.

Marie: **What advice would you give to others hoping to increase access to lactation services for women of color?**

Sherry: Be creative, assess your community assets, and find a way to connect what you have to what women need. When I'm considering a project large or small, I always call to mind the words of the late tennis great, Arthur Ashe, *Start where you are, use what you have, do what you can.* Finally, if you are not a woman of color yourself, join your efforts to someone who is. Allies are important to the cause, but they must take their lead from someone who is a member of a community of color. At Uzazi Village, we counsel many allies around the state and around the country to place women of color in central roles when doing outreaches to communities of color. On our website, you'll find the success stories (Uzazi Champions) of those we have worked with to improve lactation rates in other communities of color.

Acknowledgment:
We were successful in finding a hospital that would partner with us in allowing our interns to do mentorship hours with their IBCLCs at their facility: North Kansas City Hospital, 2800 Clay Edwards Drive, North Kansas City, MO 64116. Reprinted from the Lactation Matters blog, April 17, 2014. Used with permission.

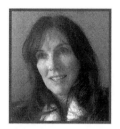

Marie Hemming, IBCLC, RLC, is the mother of three breastfed children (now 20, 16, and 15 years of age). She developed and taught a 20-hour breastfeeding class at the Florida School of Traditional Midwifery. She is currently volunteering as an IBCLC, RLC, and lay community counselor at Birthline of San Diego, CA, serving families living in poverty.

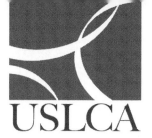

Reflections on Lactation in the African American Community

Kathi Barber, BS, CLEC[1]

Keywords: African-American, cultural competency, culture

Lactation advocacy, promotion, and counseling has undergone a number of changes in the African American community. From programs funded by the government to contemplative reviews of the business of lactation, the breastfeeding rates of Black women have made an unhurried increase. With straightforward acumen, Kathi Barber shares her reflections on working in the field.

As I look back over my experience in the field of lactation, it's hard to fathom that I have been in the business of breastfeeding advocacy and counseling for more than 15

1 writekb@gmail.com, Owner, SimplyCreativa; Founder of African American Breastfeeding Alliance

years. When I started this journey back in 2000, the idea of an organization to promote breastfeeding and provide lactation support to African American women was new, different, and long overdue. Today, the need is as strong as it ever was, and I have seen a distinct evolution in the promotion of breastfeeding to Black women.

The profession of lactation in general has grown by leaps and bounds. When I was trained as a breastfeeding peer counselor (BPC), there were but a few, and those who were employed largely worked for the Women, Infants, and Children (WIC) program. Now, BPCs are trained throughout the spectrum of healthcare settings.

The number of professionals with the International Board Certified Lactation Consultant credential has also increased exponentially, although too few are employed by hospitals and fewer still are African American. Today, more people understand what "lactation" means and that there is someone, other than an obstetrician or pediatrician, to actually call for breastfeeding support. Breastfeeding has never been more advertised, discussed, and cajoled in the media than in recent years.

Yet breastfeeding rates in the African American community are still much too low. The upside? Initiation rates have increased. The downside? Compared to all the work that has been done, from the individual practitioner to government campaigns, the rates have inched along much too slowly. When I stop to consider why strides to improve breastfeeding rates in the African American community have resulted in minimal, large-scale results, it's a bit of a quandary, but just a bit.

When I founded the African American Breastfeeding Alliance (AABA) in 2000, breastfeeding promotion for Black women was consigned to the following:

» WIC breastfeeding support

» One Anita Baker–sponsored WIC video

» Outdated photos

» La Leche League breastfeeding peer counselor program

There were no websites, blogs, brochures, newsletters, or campaigns targeting breastfeeding in the African American community.

In fact, the issue of breastfeeding and African American women was but a small blip on the public health scene. I have watched *Breastfeeding and African American Women* ebb and flow, along with funding to support the cause. *The Blueprint for Action on Breastfeeding,* published by the Department of Health and Human Services (HHS), and championed by former Surgeon General, Dr. David Satcher, encouraged support of breastfeeding in communities of color. Then, and now, most lactation research studies focus on Black mothers from the WIC or low-income populations. Women outside of WIC or other government-subsidized programs may never be exposed to any these important breastfeeding resources. There is a miniscule number of research and recorded data that takes into account the nuances of Black women from Middle America, those women with incomes above the poverty line to middle-income status. These women we know are rarely, if ever, researched on any social, economic, or social level. You have to wonder—how do the breastfeeding rates, practices, and beliefs of middle- and upper-class Black women factor into the true picture of breastfeeding in the African American Community?

Over the past 15 years, many lactation practitioners, organizations, and government agencies have championed the importance of breastfeeding, supporting breastfeeding, increasing breastfeeding rates, as well as strategies to improve breastfeeding among African American women and their families. National advertising campaigns, national statewide coalitions, panel discussion at conferences, and even the celebrities breastfeeding have shed light on this important topic. However, at the grassroots, community level among African American women in the birth world, breastfeeding has been a burgeoning health issue that has never ebbed.

I firmly believe the answer to any problem comes from within the very source of the problem at hand. The hindrance to a dramatic shift in African American breastfeeding rates is three-fold: the breastfeeding politic, organizational sustainability, and our approach to lactation promotion. From *Milk, Money, and Madness: The Culture and Politics of Breastfeeding* (Baumslag & Michels, 1995), we viewed a glimpse of breastfeeding politics as it related to infant formula, society, history, economics, healthcare, and parenting. The breastfeeding politics I'm referring to is the collection of organizations and agencies that have been at the helm of all breastfeeding policy, promotion, and campaigns, and that have crafted the professional standards and lactation *issues of the day*. These groups have been well-meaning and successful in the way the profession, and largely the society, looks at lactation. Still, Black breastfeeding rates remain the lowest in the country.

Until very recently, African American organizations have not been leading the overall lactation health campaign for our own community. We've been at the table—as partners and collaborators, but when it comes to creating standards of practice for breastfeeding in the African American community, we have not been the captains of our own ship. We are invited to meetings and consulted on projects, yet our organizations have not had the financial sustainability, like our colleagues, to manage programs and make monumental change. There is no need to name the breastfeeding powers that be—that's for another article.

There is a severe lack of cultural understanding from lactation professionals interacting with Black moms. I've been leading workshops for professionals over the last 15 years. It's the primary reason I wrote my second book on lactation management and African American moms.

The fact that I have been speaking on lactation and cultural competency, inequity in lactation and communities of color and other similar topics—no these are not new phrases—for more than 15 years shows that we have a long way to go in the profession. If we can't be internally proactive and confront inequities at the organizational level within lactation, how can we expect to effect change at the level of mothers?

Still … It's exciting to watch all the changes, ups, and downs, as well as challenges that exist among my peers who are in this labor of love. Perhaps if we shift our perspective, decipher a sustainable funding stream, and give our old approach to breastfeeding promotion a face-lift, breastfeeding in the African American community will no longer be an issue to target, but a positive change to reflect on.

Reference

Baumslag, N., & Michels, D. L. (1995). *Milk, money, and madness: The culture and politics of breastfeeding.* Westport, CT: Greenwood Publishing.

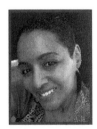 **Kathi Barber** is the author of *The Black Woman's Guide to Breastfeeding: The Definitive Guide to Nursing for African American Mothers* and *Lactation Management: Strategies for Working with African American Moms. The Black Woman's Guide to Breastfeeding* is a "how-to" breastfeeding book that focuses on the specific challenges that Black mothers face. Kathi's second book, *Lactation Management*, provides guidance to lactation and other professionals who need assistance in effectively working with their African American clients. Kathi founded the

AABA in January of 2000. AABA, a nonprofit organization that worked to educate African American women and families about the importance of breastfeeding, was the first organization to promote and support breast-feeding in Black communities. By creating a groundswell of interest, the AABA successfully mobilized women, groups, and agencies across the country to focus on the singular needs of breastfeeding in this community.

Kathi travels across the country to speak and to train peer counselors, and educate clinical and paraprofessional staff on promoting and supporting breastfeeding in the African American community. She has consulted with the U.S. HHS and a host of other organizations on this important topic. Her work has been featured in *The Washington Post, Ebony Magazine, USA Today,* and the *Chicago Tribune*; on the National Public Radio (NPR); and many other media outlets.

Beyond breastfeeding advocacy, Kathi supports women in the area of depression. Currently, she is writing her third book on women of color and mental health. Her work has forged a passion and commitment to social justice and equal rights for reproductive, birth, and overall health in communities of color and other groups society has placed on the fringe! Most important to know about Kathi is that she is an outrageously proud mother of two teenagers.

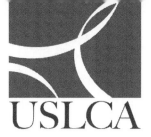

Additional Organizations That Address Health Inequities Within the African American Community

Kathleen Kendall-Tackett, PhD, IBCLC, RLC, FAPA[1]

Keywords: Breastfeeding, African Americans, Black mothers, community organizations

The increase in breastfeeding rates in the African American community is largely due to the efforts of several grassroots organizations. This article briefly describes some of these organizations, highlighting their objectives, mission, founders, and beginnings.

The Black Mothers' Breastfeeding Association

The Black Mothers' Breastfeeding Association (BMBFA) is based in Detroit, Michigan. Kiddada Green is the founding

---

1   kkendallt@gmail.com

executive director (Figure 1). Their vision is to make positive cultural sentiments about breastfeeding and multigenerational breastfeeding support within African American families and communities.

The mission of the BMBFA is to "reduce racial inequities in breastfeeding support for African Americans by building foundational networks of support, and strengthening systems to overcome historical, societal, and social barriers to breastfeeding success." Their goal is to reduce national rates of racial disparities in lower rates of breastfeeding in African Americans. They want to accomplish their goal by providing education and support to African Americans and the agencies that serve them.

Explore the website at http://blackmothersbreastfeeding.org/ or contact them at BlackMothersBreastfeeding@gmail.com

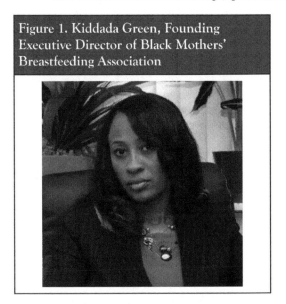

Figure 1. Kiddada Green, Founding Executive Director of Black Mothers' Breastfeeding Association

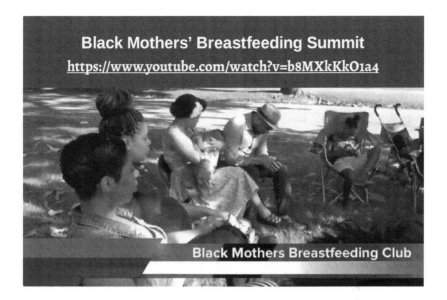

Reaching Our Sisters Everywhere

Reaching Our Sisters Everywhere (ROSE), Inc., http:// www.breastfeedingrose.org/, was founded in July 2011 by three Atlanta-based women who have worked in the field of maternal and child health for the past 25 years. Kimarie Bugg, MSN, FNP-BC, MPH, CLC, observed how the prenatal healthcare system not only failed to teach and encourage breastfeeding, but also often impeded it.

ROSE's initiatives include:

a. improving access to breastfeeding in the African American community,

b. reclaiming their breastfeeding experience, and

c. reforming healthcare through breastfeeding.

Since its founding, ROSE has grown to a network that includes physicians, nurses, nutritionists, social workers, peer counselors, and parents (Figure 2). ROSE seeks to enhance, encourage, support, promote, and protect breastfeeding throughout the U.S. by working to reduce the breastfeeding disparities among African American women, and to strengthen the health of their babies and families through mentoring, training, breastfeeding support groups, social support, outreach, education, legislation, health policies, and social marketing.

ROSE's primary goal is to increase the percentage of African American women who breastfeed and thereby reach the target breastfeeding goal outlined in *Healthy People* 2020. To achieve the 81% increase of African American women who breastfeed by 2020, there will need to be nationally focused programs that involve a range of stakeholders: breastfeeding women, individuals, family, healthcare providers, and community and public policymakers.

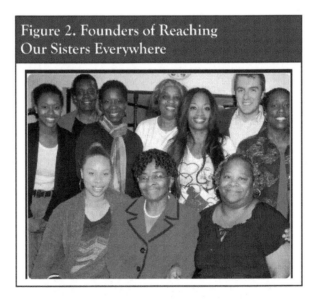

Figure 2. Founders of Reaching Our Sisters Everywhere

A More Excellent Way

Monique Sims-Harper, DrPH, MPH, RD, CLE (Figure 3), is the chief executive officer and founder of A More Excellent Way Health Improvement Organization (MEW). This project came about as part Dr. Sims's dissertation project at the University of California at Berkeley. Her dissertation title was, *Engaging the Faith Community to Improve the Breastfeeding Rates of African American Women*. MEW was formed in 2005 and incorporated in December of 2007. Dr. Sims partnered with her church, Revival Center Ministries, in pioneering the MEW Breastfeeding Project, which consisted of conducting focus groups that informed a church-placed infant feeding and parenting training and intervention.

The first MEW peer counselor training and baby shower was successful in training 14 breastfeeding peer counselors in the art and practice of breastfeeding support and ministering to more than 100 men and women. The training and baby shower have been repeated at several churches in Solano County, including True Love Baptist Church and Tabernacle of David Missionary Baptist Church. The plan is to continue to train leaders in the community to improve Solano County's breastfeeding rates, particularly among African Americans. This project intends to improve the health and survival of African American infants.

The organization aims to promote wellness and reduce health disparities. MEW engages the community, and particularly churches, to provide health education, information, and resources.

Figure 3. Monique Sims-Harper, Founder and CEO of A More Excellent Way

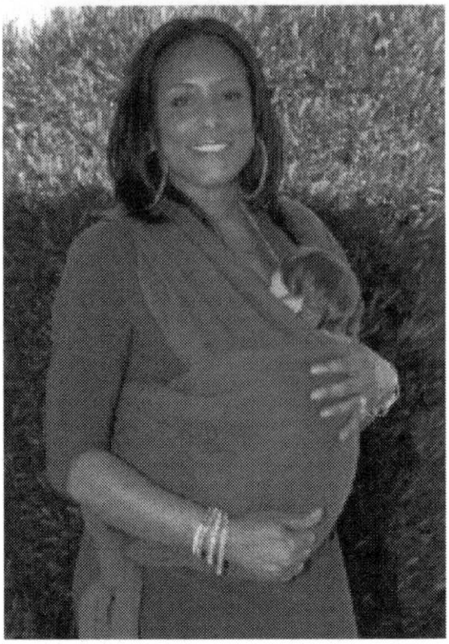

Since our organization began, the rates of African American breastfeeding have increased significantly. However, the African American and White gap in breastfeeding rates still persists. Our goal is to eliminate this disparity in breastfeeding and that 75% of African American women in Solano County & Contra Costa County breastfeed their babies for at least one year.

Dr. Sims is the proud mother of two breastfed sons and one foster daughter, and is guardian to her three nephews. Dr. Sims is also a registered dietitian who has a passion for improving the nutrition and health of her family and community. You can contact Monique at monique@mewpeers.org or http://www.mewpeers.org/.

Blacktating

Elita Kalma, CLC, is the founder of the popular blog, Blacktating (Figure 4). She started her blog to get answers to her questions about breastfeeding. She was hoping to find another mother out there at 4 in the morning who was also breastfeeding and perhaps had questions of her own. But she noticed that she was never hearing back from other mothers of color, even when she specifically looked for them. She wanted to know where the other Black breastfeeding moms were and how could she connect with them. When her son was 4 months old, she decided to start Blacktating. The blog has given her a way to reach other mothers of color, and it has caught the eye of the professional community who wants to know more about the breastfeeding experiences of African American women.

> My goal used to be to just get people outside of my family to read my blog, but now my dream is to become an International Board Certified Lactation Consultant, and write a parenting book for moms of color who are interested in natural and attachment parenting.

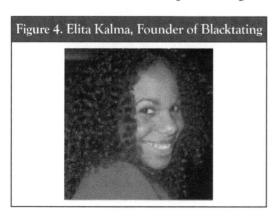

Figure 4. Elita Kalma, Founder of Blacktating

Elita's blog can be found at http://blacktating.blogspot.com/

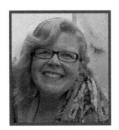 **Kathleen Kendall-Tackett, PhD, IBCLC, RLC, FAPA,** is a health psychologist, International Board Certified Lactation Consultant, and the owner and editor-in-chief of *Praeclarus Press*, a small press specializing in women's health. Dr. Kendall-Tackett is editor-in-chief of *Clinical Lactation*, fellow of the American Psychological Association (APA) in Health and Trauma Psychology, past-president of the APA Division of Trauma Psychology, and editor-in-chief of *Psychological Trauma*.

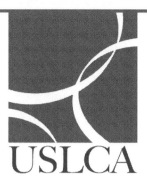

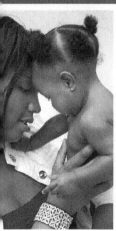
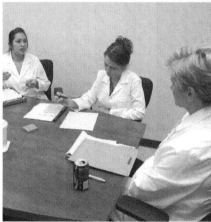
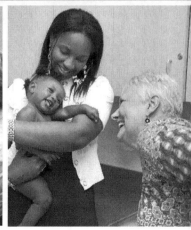

The U.S. Lactation Consultant Association Presents
Clinical Lactation Monographs

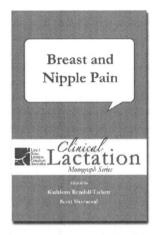
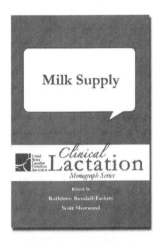

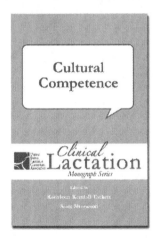
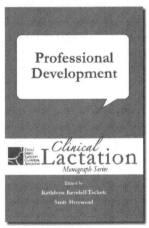

Praeclarus Press
Excellence in Women's Health

www.PraeclarusPress.com

Breastfeeding Titles from Praeclarus Press

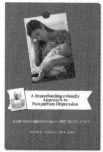

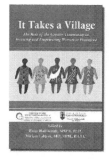

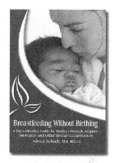

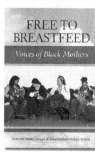

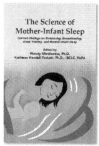

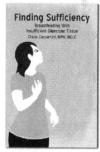

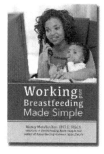

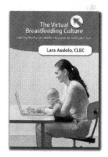

Praeclarus Press
Excellence in Women's Health

www.PraeclarusPress.com

Made in the USA
San Bernardino, CA
07 June 2017